MS Won't Get Me Down:
Facts, Info and Encouragements for MS Persons and Their Caregivers

by Elvira Heiser James

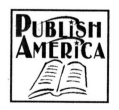

PublishAmerica
Baltimore

First printing

ISBN: 1-4137-4985-2
PUBLISHED BY PUBLISHAMERICA, LLLP
www.publishamerica.com
Baltimore

Printed in the United States of America

Foreword to First Edition

There are some good books on the market that talk about multiple sclerosis, what it is and how to live with it, but I found something missing in them. They were either too technical, focusing too narrowly on a fraction of the big picture, were filled with case histories or were too biographical for my taste. With *MS Won't Get Me Down*, I want to present a comprehensive work of information, clarifications and explanations, presented in layperson's terms. The reader will also find suggestions for living, references, hints and encouragements for the person who has MS. In addition, I want to include the caregivers, the people who love and care for somebody who has MS and would like to know what the MS person goes through.

This book is a partial reprint of some of the newsletters I wrote for the Crawford (Ohio) County MS Support Group during the years of 1988 to 1993. I have added new material and deleted what was only of local interest or what would violate the confidence I have been entrusted with over the years.

Some of this material, for instance "The ABC of MS," has been reprinted in Relay, the Northwest Ohio Chapter of the MS Society's official newsletter and one piece, titled "Others Who Know...Others Who Care" has been adopted by the Chapter as official literature.

Some Points I'd Like to Stress:

1. All conclusions, interpretations and opinions are mine, unless something is attributed to a specific author, speaker or writer.

2. I am no doctor and did not consult with one for this book. If you discover misinterpretations or what you perceive as errors, I apologize. I do not give medical advice, just report what I read, tell you what our speakers said and how I interpret it, talk about what I am doing or what I am taking to ease my life. Thus, please do check out everything that pertains to medical theory and practice with your physician or other health care provider.

3. I do believe most people who have MS do not consider themselves patients. (I will explain later what brought that discovery on.) For this reason, I will use the terms people who have MS, MS persons or MSers. I have played around with some other shorthand symbols, but they came too close to PMS, and I did not want to indicate that I might be talking about a different group of sufferers.

4. You might discover what you perceive as misrepresentations from the beginning pages to later ones. The reason for this is the fact that research and assorted MS facts change quite frequently and quickly, and since I'm a compulsive revisionist (in other words, I'm never satisfied with my work and revise heavily), they really creep up on me. I do dislike retyping continually but want to include the new info-ergo the apparent discrepancies.

5. I believe strongly that thinking is one of the most important activities one can engage in. I find it plays an enormous, awesome, even terrifying role in determining how we act, react and interact with ourselves and others. That is the reason why I would like to invite you right from the start to do a lot of thinking.

6. There is one thing I have trouble with, and that is writing for long in a formal style—you know with "For's" beginning each fourth sentence. That's why I wrote my newsletter and why I write my other non-fiction works in an informal style, sort of like holding a talk with a friend.

I also like to play around with words and, as attention-getters, present sentences ungrammatically. I found this method extremely helpful in getting my kids' attention while raising them.

I'll end this foreword the way I end all my correspondence to MS persons: Best wishes for permanent remission.

—Elvie

Foreword to the Second Edition

With the help of my husband and a generous printer, I compiled the pages of the first edition of *MS Won't Get Me Down* in 1996 and gave about a dozen copies to interested people. Since then, research has discovered multiple sclerosis. These years have also brought four specifically-designed-for-MS medications on the market, the ABCs (Avonex, Betaseron and Copaxon) and R (Rebif), which were speedily approved by the Food and Drug Administration. For these reasons, I have decided to update this manuscript. Also, thanks to research, updated news has become available. Someone may point out that a check of book lists at Amazon.com or Barnes and Noble's shelves shows there are quite a few books about MS already available—why add another one? In fact, yesterday (15 November 2003) I checked the Barnes and Noble website and discovered that their listing includes 458 books pertaining to MS.

Although my words from the first edition's foreword still apply, namely that I am somewhat uncomfortable with the books I have read. I appreciate the theory, but as I said, I missed something. It is difficult to define, but I believe it shows that most of the authors didn't have multiple sclerosis themselves and their words lack a certain feeling tone, sensitivity, sincerity—I don't find the right words to describe it; it is just a vague feeling of something missing. I don't want to boast about my knowledgeability, but I have been told that some books are just too technical to be understood by laypersons.

In a third category of books, there are those with an abundance of histories—and I do dislike them intensely.

For all these reasons I envisioned presenting a comprehensive book where a lot of material appears in one place, writing it from the standpoint of one layperson to another. I have also been told that readers of my newsletter and the first compilation of this information appreciated the humor in and the informality of my writing, and so I decided to keep it that way.

Now a few words of explanations:

1. About MS acceptance. I mentioned MS acceptance on one of the bulletin boards and received some strong words of chastisement, declaring that the writers would never accept having MS because they considered that as passively giving up.

That is a wrong interpretation of my words. My concept of acceptance is based on reality perception. Something like, I have multiple sclerosis; I accept that as a given and devise a way to live my life in a manner which is productive, doing the best I can do while realizing and honoring my limits. Attaining this acceptance brings on peace of mind, soul and spirit, helps to be strong, doing what we can do without overdoing. In this way, we can be the best person we can be.

2. You will notice that chapter sections are separated by the letters "MSWGMD." It stands for MS won't get me down. This sentence plus "I won't give up," "I won't let it (MS, life, trouble, etc.) get me down" and "God helps those who help themselves" are my life truisms, my mantra, my battle cry.

Allow me to end this chapter on a lighter note.

Throughout this book you will hear me talk about instances of me having changed my I'll never...to an I did...Here is one non-MS-related example.

For years, my son-in-law, the computer whizzzzz, had nagged me to get a computer, which supposedly would increase my output and make my life soooohhh much easier. Well, this stubborn Taurus said no, nope and never!!! Well, that rascal (the son-in-law) and my daughter came over to my house one evening, carrying that contraption called a computer, with her carrying keyboard and cables. He, without saying a word, removed my word processor from my desk, put that thing in its place and expertly hooked it up. One of them (I think it was my daughter) said soothingly, "Now, Mami, if you can't hack it, we'll take it back and get you your word processor back." (I suppose she didn't use those exact words, but that's what I heard.)

Ha! Nobody tells me I can't hack something without me giving it one darn good try. Of course I hacked it; now I like the convenience of the bleepetybleep thing and have been upgraded four times. Since June 2000, I'm on the Internet, I happily e-mail around the world, get lots of information and participate actively on three MS Bulletin Boards.

So nobody shall ever say in my presence that old dogs can't learn new tricks or that older people lose too many brain cells to learn complex things. I'm sixty-six now and really have started living after I turned fifty and still tackle new subjects. But I swear I will stick to one "I'll never..." and that is "I'll never ever attack algebra, geometry, etc.," and that's an oath I will, shall and do plan to keep, no matter how my seventeen- (almost eighteen) year-old grandson, another computer-, science- and math-whizzzz, cajoles me.

With this book, I want to give you some material as food for thought, some tips and hints and, I hope, lots of encouragement to allow you to create a good life for yourself.

As I said above, best wishes for permanent remission.

—Elvie

P.S. To those who have read the earlier version: You will find this expanded version quite improved, different and better.

P.P.S. I revised and updated this material once more, beginning in November 2003.

P.P.P.S. And one more going-over-it in July 2004.

Chapter One
To Begin With

Introduction

Something is going on in your body, something you don't like. Do not like it at all. You have problems with your eyes, your legs or arms and hands shake, and you can't stop it, you are unsteady on your feet. You went to your family doctor, and for weeks or months, you were being sent from the eye doctor to a heart specialist, and had your liver, cholesterol and kidneys checked—with the test results coming back as being "within normal range" or something to that effect. Maybe one of them put you on arthritis medication, which didn't do a darn for you. You got impatient, feared the doctors may consider you a malingerer or hypochondriac or despaired. Finally, as a last resort, you were sent to a neurologist "for a consult."

What else but more tests. More blood tests, x-rays, evoked responses test, MRI (Magnetic Resonance Imaging) and maybe a spinal tap. If you were lucky, the doctor finally told you the tests indicate you have multiple sclerosis. Or it had been called a demyelinating disease, a neuromuscular or neurological disorder. But busy doctors (or are they uncomfortable ones) won't give you much of an explanation of what it is, what you can expect over the short or long haul, what it does to your body, you spirit or your quality of life.

13

Let me clarify why I said "If you are lucky…" Many potential MS persons hang in limbo for years. They have classical MS symptoms but no diagnosis. (If you join one or more of the MS Bulletin Boards, you will read over and over about the heartbreak of men and women with "probable or possible" MS diagnoses. The doctor says, "Since the MRI came back clean or negative, I can't make the MS diagnosis."

(I have recently read the complaints that doctors put too much credence on the MRI results and forego the so-called old-fashioned diagnostic methods [extensive neurologic testing, spinal fluid check for gamma globulin, even evoked responses tests], thus granting technology the power of diagnosis. I won't write out what the writers' conclusions were; you may easily figure out it was not very positive.)

I feel deepest sympathy with these sufferers. Isn't uncertainty worse than knowing what is going on and having something to sink one's teeth into and receive medications for—especially since experts insist the earlier one of the ABCR's are taken, the better?

MSWGMD

Now observe the person who has received a multiple sclerosis diagnosis.

Whatever it is being called, it is nothing to receive hearty congratulations for. In fact, for most people it is scary, even devastating, particularly because knowledge about the disease is so obscure.

Family members, friends, acquaintances, even half-strangers want to know what's wrong with you, why you're seeing a doctor—a neurologist at that and what does one of them specialize in—and want to know what you were in the hospital for.

The reaction you get when you do tell the truth is no help either. Unless you live in the MS Belt or a Cluster City (definitions in a moment), you will receive some blank stares. Maybe the questioner will take, even if unconsciously, a step or two away from you.

They don't know what MS is. Or they know somebody who has it, is paralyzed, totally incapacitated, unable to do anything. Thoughtlessly— or is it uncomfortably or to say something while not knowing what to say—they relate these stories. To you who has MS, it sounds as if they were relishing their tales and delight in embellishing these accounts with the goriest details of poor so-and-so's sufferings and early demise. That certainly doesn't help, except increasing anxieties, apprehensions and fears.

(I'm working at the moment on the edit of a reincarnation novel where the main character develops MS, goes through the pre-diagnosis, diagnosis and post-diagnosis stages and works herself through to a realistic view.)

No, having MS is nothing to be proud of. But neither is it something to be ashamed of. And it definitively is nothing to give up on life for.

MSWGMD

Personal reactions to the diagnosis of MS of course depend on the individual person. The following responses are the most common ones that I have observed:

People of one group give up after the diagnosis. "Why should I do anything?" they proclaim. "I'm condemned to a life of pain and suffering and probably worse. If I do something, I'll just end up a cripple faster."

Others overdo the doing, working themselves into total exhaustion to prove they're still useful individuals. Reactions resulting from these experiences are further subdivided. Those from Group A use the exhaustion as proof positive that they should not do anything from now on. Group Bers go on feeling the self-pitying martyr. Group C people talk about nothing but their illness while those from group D murmur an apologetic "I have MS." Not to forget those from group E who refuse to say anything about the MS that has them.

The healthy response, of course, would be born out of MS-acceptance, something that is not easily nor quickly achieved, given the diversity of symptoms, the different personality types of individual people and the variety of responses these individual people give.

(A hint at what *MS Won't Get Me Down* is all about. For most people, gaining MS-acceptance is a difficult process. I know. I have been there. It might take a while till you accomplish it, but it is a goal worth pursuing. Just have patience with yourself. Don't rush it. Don't talk yourself into pseudo-acceptance which your heart, mind, soul and spirit don't believe in. At first just sink your teeth into surviving. Do the most you can do without overdoing until you can say, and mean it, that there is life after an MS diagnosis, that you will live your life to the best of your abilities, do as much as you comfortably can do and that you refuse to let MS get you down. If I could help you achieve this state of equilibrium, I would be grateful.)

Now some specifics:

Diagnosis

(I use this word not to describe the process of being diagnosed with an illness but in its broader sense of analysis, overview, identification.)

I have been asked and still am being asked: "What is MS? Why doesn't one hear that much about it except when they hold fundraisers or when another actor, talk show host or politician admits to having MS?"

I'll answer the second part first because it is the easier one.

As I have already hinted at, except in the MS Belt or a Cluster city, MS is not that common an illness. The numbers of MS persons in the US stood for a long time at about 200,000 to 250,000. In March 2002, I checked on the Internet for the current statistics of diagnosed MS cases and read that the count had been upped to 250,000 to 300,000. But recently I read and hear that the numbers slowly slink upwards. Interesting, though, in January of 2004, talk show host and MSer Montel Williams visited Fox News Reporter and MSer Neil Cavuto on the *Your World* show. Among other things, Mr. Williams stated that the MS cases in America range in the 1.8 million. I found that very interesting. This may not be officially-approved numbers, but I believe he is correct.

In answer to the first part of the question, I define multiple sclerosis on the emotional level as an illness of loss of control, of uncertainties, of unpredictability. One never knows what will next happen where or when.

MS is also loneliness, fear of the future, feeling misunderstood, being attacked by fatigue and depression, helplessness and hopelessness.

But one can't expect another person to understand that, except another MSer.

Speaking on a scientific level, MS is being called an autoimmune disease; that is, a disease where the body attacks its own tissue. The immune system can no longer distinguish between foreign invaders and "the self." A viral and a genetic connection are thrown in for not-good measure.

It has been established that MS cannot start without a push. One pamphlet, printed by the National MS Society, speaks of "some unknown signal." Dr. Rammohan, from the Ohio State University MS Clinics, called it "an unknown trigger." Others speak of an "environmental trigger." I don't want to steal either of these three descriptions; I prefer to call the Big It the Factor X trigger and see this Factor X trigger as making the immune system (lately I read hint that they also start blaming the Blood Brain Barrier) get out on the wrong side of the bed, setting off MS symptoms or causing exacerbations.

Basically I explain multiple sclerosis like this: Something goes haywire in the body, aggravates Factor X trigger. It snakes up to the immune system, urging it to chomp away on our precious myelin, causing an inflammation. (Myelin is the fatty sheathing around nerve fibers in the white, the myelinated matter, of the brain.) The holes, called lesions, where the myelin sheath is eaten away are covered by scar tissues, the MS plaques. In turn, the orders from the brain can no longer be smoothly relayed to the muscles of the various body parts, and that causes the MS symptoms.

This, simplistically, can be likened to an ordinary electric cord. If something has burned a hole in the insulation or the plug is wobbly, you can plug the utensil in, but it won't brew you a pot of coffee or, as I said during high school presentations, it won't play your boombox.

Up to 1985, (I think it was around that time; some thief sneaks around, steals my time and I can't keep track of it) an MS diagnosis was a hit-and-miss affair. The doctor nodded wisely or gravely and said: "Well, since it isn't this and can't be that and doesn't look like something else, it might be multiple sclerosis." Nowadays, doctors have more precise tools and in most cases can say: "It is MS."

The most accurate diagnostic tool is the MRI. I don't know how it works; all I know is that it works, showing the MS lesions. Yes, there are still many people, as I have already mentioned, who complain bitterly that they have all the right symptoms but don't get a definitive diagnosis.

The Symptoms

The National MS Society calls one of the MS stages "relapsing-remitting," but I prefer the old definitions of "exacerbation and remission." It's much clearer, and even others know the meaning of these terms, don't you think?

Symptoms are, as one doctor defined it, "as diverse as the individual MS patient." These symptoms range from endurable to leaving the person somewhat impaired to being incapacitated.

Some people don't even know they have MS. They only feel some mild discomfort or have a few flare-ups which are diagnosed as something else, a sprain or strain or thinking they have caught a cold or have a touch of arthritis. For most of us MSers though, those afflicted with the exacerbation-remission type, flare-ups come and go at their pleasure, stay a while and go away for a while, but even after they go, they often leave the affected body part a little weaker. In other words, it's up and down the unpredictability ladder as doled out at our body's discretion. During the remission we feel relatively all-rightish till the next bout hits up and down and down and up, like ascending and descending a spiral staircase at dizzying speeds.

Specifically speaking, the major MS symptoms are:

- Numbness, stiffness, clumsiness, things slip out of fingers.
- The spasticity-tremors, the limbs—most notably the legs—shake and tremble uncontrollably.
- The cognitive dysfunctions—memory loss or impairment, inability to concentrate or focus, trying to think of the proper word which

won't appear on the mind's surface, not remembering how to do simple things, (I have heard Msers complain about not remembering what they have to do, how to cook or work the compute, you know, being unable to do something that used to be done automatically.)

- Slowed, slurred, halting, monotonous speech patterns.
- Optic neuritis, also called the first sign of a potential MS affliction— blurred or double vision, temporary loss of vision, particularly in one eye, vision clouded as if one had a gray veil before one's eyes.
- All sorts of bowel and bladder problems.
- No strength or a feeling of heaviness in a limb, having trouble lifting the coffee cup, let alone the whole pot, because the hand shakes so bad. (I mention coffee so often because my mother-in-law made a coffeeholic out of me.)
- The pins and needles sensation, feeling as if the hand, arm, foot or leg had "fallen asleep."
- Unsteadiness, loss of balance, knees or ankles buckling under and giving out.
- Especially bothersome is that dratted fatigue which comes out of nowhere and zaps all strength. It can strike any time of the day—or night, if you are a shift worker—and you can't do anything but close your eyes.

Nobody can predict when an exacerbation will strike, how severe it will be, which area will be affected, how long exacerbation or remission will last or how devastating the attack will be this time.

Are you declaring that with all the advances available to science, researchers should have made faster inroads by now?

Well, I grant them a little benefit of doubt. As I will explain, MS is a complicated disease. Consider this: Billions of nerve fibers (and that's no exaggeration), chosen at random, can be demyelinated, and the affected body part cannot function properly. This brings on the widest variety of exacerbation symptoms of differing severity during an exacerbation. They stop, or at least become less incapacitating, during a spontaneous remission. Add to that the wide scope of the field needing to be investigated (remember immune system, neurologic, viral and genetic), and you can picture why the research is such a long, drawn-out process before researchers come up with specific, factual answers. Additionally, we have to face the fact that MS is not one of the so-called glamorous diseases nor one that affects a large group of people like heart disease, cancer, AIDS, Parkinson's or Alzheimer's. And we don't have powerful spokespersons lobbying for us.

The most difficult to accept and cope with is the chronic-progressive type of MS. Thank God not too many people are hit with this fast-advancing one.

Facts

In 1996, I had written: "Some facts have been conclusively established..." On March 9, 2002, I checked *www.personalhealthzone.com* on the Internet. Reading their material proved that these facts still hold true and not much has been added to it.

And no surprise to us MSers, nothing significant has changed or improved now, toward the end of 2003.

Following, then, are the facts as outlined in 1996:

- MS begins between the ages of ten to sixty years, with the average lying between twenty and forty. That is why MS is being called the illness of young adults.
- Diagnostic age does not equal onset age. A person can have MS for many years before it is being diagnosed as such.
- More women than men contract MS. Ladies, let's scream discrimination!
- Factors that may start the active disease process, aggravate symptoms or precipitate exacerbations: Heat and humidity, general poor health, psychological trauma, emotional or physical stress
- Stress: Some sources insist stress does not cause flare-ups, while others say it is so responsible for attacks. My money is with the second group. I say stress definitively plays a major role in multiple sclerosis.
- MS per se does not shorten the life span significantly. We had all ages represented in our support group—people as young as twenty-two and others who were in their sixties, and the older ones were

still doing well. (In April 2002, I read in our local newspaper that one of our former members had died at age seventy-five, and as far as I know, he was still getting around till shortly before his death.)

- MS can strike any part of the body connected with the central nervous system.
- Most MS persons have to cope with fatigue and spasticity. (Nowadays I add depression to it.)
- It is being said that seventy-five percent of MSers are only minimally or moderately impaired; through adjustments, they can lead productive lives.

In 2002, as well as November 2003, I can repeat that there is still no cure near the horizon, but the ABCs (Avonex, Betaseron and Copaxone, plus since 9 March 2002, Rebif) have been approved by the FDA for prescription in the United States. These injectables are designed to help shorten or decrease the numbers of exacerbations. Oral medications are also available to ease an MSer's life. Specifics later on.

The MS Belt

This is the name given to an imaginary line separating MS-prone areas from areas where one is less likely to find a preponderance of MS cases. People living above that line are more likely to have MS than those living below the line.

In the late 1980s, Mr. Michael Wood, a reporter with the newspaper *Toledo Blade* (Ohio) wrote an excellent article, factual yet sensitive, on MS. He defined the MS Belt as a line drawn from Newport News, Virginia to Santa Cruz, California. Here in Ohio, MS incidents are at their highest in the northern counties. Around the world, this north equals highest MS occurrences holds also true.

It's Not Inherited...

...or so they proclaim.

For quite some time, those who compile statistics and give them out as facts have said that it is unlikely that a person could develop MS just because a close relative has or had MS. The percentages that it could happen was placed quite low—somewhere in the single digits. Although the numerical values have risen steadily over the years, scientists are still not ready to grudgingly admit to more than the susceptibility factor…blah blah blah.

Well, it has been undeniably established that autoimmune diseases run in families. Okay, it has also been given out as a fact that multiple sclerosis is an autoimmune disease—so what can that mean but that it, too, runs in families?

That does not surprise me. I'm no scientist, but, I mean, come on, we have learned in elementary school that each child receives genes from both father and mother, and if one of the parents carries the faulty genes which are in part responsible for MS, it is more than likely that the genes are passed on to proud offsprings of the parents and that the Factor X trigger will be activated in at least some of them.

Well, let them learned heads tell us what they want; we who have MS and have family members who have or had MS, we know better.

MSWGMD

In 1982, when I was diagnosed, it was easy to explain multiple sclerosis—not much was known about it. In 1990, I put together a fact sheet and major research paper for our support group which started with the following two paragraphs:

> We don't know why a lot of things happen—nobody knows what causes MS, nobody can predict severity or duration of an exacerbation, nobody can foretell how fast or how slow disabilities will advance, nobody has a cure for MS.
>
> Yes, it is frightening, this living at the mercy of one's body, never knowing for sure what will happen next and then what and what after that. In other words, an MS person can't really plan or schedule anything, especially not long-range.

As I said, I typed these two paragraphs in 1990, and they were true then. In March of 2002, these same facts were true, and in November 2003, not much had significantly been added to or taken away from those sentences. And you know something? Today is 9 July 2004, and these facts are still as true now as they were then.

But even if you are a fairly newly diagnosed MSer, don't fling this book away, believing the situation is hopeless. It is not. Over the last decade, some inroads have been made toward finding cause and maybe even a cure. The ABCRs have gained FDA approval, and other medications are in the hopper. I'll talk about that later.

It is a fact that scientists all over the world are digging in and working on several fronts to wrest some secrets off MS. They consider the theory of the sneaky, long-acting virus hiding somewhere in the body—but where in the body and which specific virus and how it enters the body is still conjecture. They have made some strides toward discovering why the immune system is out of whack and doesn't know any longer what and whom to protect and what to destroy. Studies concerning the flawed genes aspect have been particularly successful and the Blood Brain Barrier research is out of the baby shoes stages too. Despite extensive studies, there is still not much known about the Factor X trigger. Personally, I believe in the end they will discover that all the features will interplay in explaining, preventing and curing MS.

And that, fitting all the pieces together to form a cohesive whole, that, I believe is the most onerous task.

Glossary

The following is a list of words you might run into in articles or books (this one included), hear them tossed out in speeches or have health care professionals verbalize them. You, in order of not wanting to risk sounding—uh, let's call it unsophisticated—don't want to publicly ask the meaning of. (Pretty unsophisticated sentence structure, I know, but you did understand what I meant though, right?)

But please do remember, these are unscientific definitions by a layperson, presented in layperson's terms. For professional information, ask your doctor, nurse or other health care professional.

Antibodies: Immune system term. They are created to fight the intruders. In MS though, they think the myelin is the invader and needs to be destroyed.

Antigen: Immune system term. The anti means that they are against us. They have markings on them that identify them as bad guys.

Ataxia: Being unsteady on one's feet, being unable to properly coordinate our movements. It attacks mainly the walking or the movement of the arms.

Autoimmune Disease: Diseases where the body can't distinguish between "self" and "non-self," that is, illnesses where the body attacks itself.

Axon: See next section, the brain discussion.

Blood-brain Barrier: It is a membrane that shields the brain from junk that swims in the blood (white blood cells for instance) from infiltrating the brain. In MS, the blood-brain barrier is leaky and does let the Myelin Basic Proteins debris into the inner sanctum where it has no business being. (I have read in October/November 2003 that researchers find this area important and are actively investigating it. That's why I add it to immune system, genetics and viral theory as significant.)

B Cells: They kinda go along with the T-cells. They are more immune system terms. The B cells are born in the bone marrow and fight foreign invaders.

Braces: They help prevent falls through steadying ankles and knees, keep the toes from curling under and causing falls. The ones with air cushions are more comfortable than the hard plastic ones. (I can attest to that from experience; I had the hard plastic type and can't wear them any longer because my feet have grown wider.)

Clonus: A sign that muscles contract when they are not supposed to.

Contracture: A decrease in the range of motion in a muscle due to stiffness.

Cytokine: They're the troublemakers, siccing the T-cells to start the attack work on the wrong matter—the myelin—and bringing about the inflammation which brings about the scarring which brings about the multifarious sclerosing (scarring, lesions) which brings about the exasperating symptoms which bring about our misery.

Dendrites: See next section, the brain discussions.

Diplopia: A sign of optic neuritis. It's double vision.

Dysarthria: Slurred speech.

Exacerbation: A flare-up, attack, new MS symptoms appear or old ones get more aggravating. One speaker called them exasperations, which is quite fitting.

EAE: (Experimental Allergic Encephalomyelitis) Inflammation and demyelination in animals, particularly mice, which mimics our MS symptoms. A great assist in research projects. Can bring greatly satisfying results if PETA (that animal rights group) lets scientists continue their work. These scientists induced EAE in the animals by making them sick through injecting myelin basic protein. The protein causes the animal's immune system to attack the nervous system, and in turn, special medications try to improve the condition of the mice which will eventually, hopefully, lead to medications which can improve the condition of human MS persons.

Fatigue: A tiredness affecting most MS persons. It hits unexpectedly, zaps all strength and can come on as early as five minutes after waking up from a refreshing sleep.

Immune System: It is supposed to keep us healthy by getting rid of new and old foes—bacteria, viruses, fungi, protozoa or whatever they're called. It wants to do a good job and keep its life-giver healthy. Eagerly it sticks its armies—the T and B cells—to attack what it sees as invading health robbers. Well, in its enthusiasm, or if the system is deceived and doesn't know right from wrong, the macrophages and lymphocytes happily attack the myelin, not realizing that they do a harmful job by gobbling up what the host needs to stay healthy. (You suppose the immune system at least feels guilt, shame and remorse? Naw, I doubt it; it probably is proud of its work.)

Immunoglobulin or Gamma Immunoglobulin: Another part of the immune system and an aid in diagnosing MS. During the diagnostic procedure, the doctor tests the cerebrospinal fluid via a spinal tap for the presence of immunoglobulins—which in MS persons is elevated. I remember that my neurologist told me my immunoglobulin was high, and based on that, plus the evoked responses test along with the findings of the inclusive neurological exams, he made my MS diagnosis.

Incontinence: Bladder trouble, being unable to void, creates the need to catheterize; or having to go when one has to go.

Lesions: Another word for the scarring of MS plagues.

Lymphocytes: Immune system term. White blood cells, signifying that an infection is going on somewhere.

Myelin: The fatty substance covering the axons, the so-called white matter of the brain, to smooth and speed up the travel orders from the brain to the muscles.

Myelin Basic Protein: When the T-cells gnaw away on the myelin, little shards or shavings fall off. Combined with white blood cells that eventually shows up in the spinal fluid. It's interesting, when that myelin basic protein is injected in laboratory mice, they develop EAE, an MS-like illness.

Neuron: The basic nerve cell with attached axon, dendrite and synapse.

Nystagmus: Another sign of optic neuritis; jerky eye movement, blurred vision.

Oligoclonal Bands: Another antibody protein which shows up in the spinal fluid.

Oligodentrocytes: (Oligos for short) These are the cells which manufacture the myelin. Major research concentrates on how the oligos can be nudged into remyelinating the damaged nerve fibers.

Optic Neuritis: Inflammation of the optic nerve. My ophthalmologist told me when he sees a patient with optic neuritis, he would like to send her or him to a neurologist because it is often the first sign of pending MS. (But of course he is not allowed to. You know, the principle of the union janitor not being allowed to install the light bulb.)

Pain: If someone tells you, "If it hurts, it ain't MS," don't believe 'em. There is pain associated with MS—sharp stabs which I call insect bites on the inside of my body, and there is the well-known face pain and other physical hurts.

Paraparesis: Partial paralysis, usually affecting the lower limbs.

Parestesia: The sensation of a limb being asleep, that tingling, pins-and-needles sensation in different parts of the body.

Plaques: The areas where the myelin has been devoured. They are scar tissue, which hinder the nerve impulses from travelling easy, smooth and quick—and under normal circumstances, they fly at mach speed. Just imagine you want to wiggle your big toe and before you even have finished that thought the action is completed. Now that is speedy.

Receptors: They're the lock-and-key proteins on the cell surface to let the right antigen or T-cell find out where it should go.

Remission: That blessed state of feeling relatively symptom-free, when we feel fairly good, when no new symptoms appear; the time between the last and the next flare-up.

Spasticity: That, the same as fatigue, is another cross most of us MSers have to bear. Outward signs: Spasms, stiffness, tightness hindering the muscles' smooth functioning and movement, jerky motions, tremors, shaking of the limb—and that can be deeply embarrassing when you sit at your kids' ballgame, holler a praise to your kid who has just made that excellent game-saving deed and suddenly your legs start shaking violently and for the life of you, you can't stop it. Or your hands shake so badly that you can barely hold the coffee cup. Or it could be that you put more wrong than right letters on the computer screen because the hand has a mind of its own.

Synapse: See next section, the brain discussions.

T-cells: Another party of the immune system. The same as B cells, they are lymphocytes, just produced in different parts of the body. They come in different sub-categories—killer, helper and suppressor T-cells are the major ones. They ferret the intruder out, eliminate it with all kinds of proteins and chemicals, and when the job is done, the suppressor T-cells say: "We're done with this one for the moment. Stop producing any more." But, uh, like kids, they don't always listen too well.

White Matter: The myelinated axons.

Weakness: A heaviness of an arm or legs, easy fatigability, unable to use that body part effectively and efficiently as you could in pre-MS times. Loss or lack of strength.

The Brain

I have often been asked about the brain and would like to provide some definition of words and concepts. Here, too, please keep in mind that I'm no expert and can only give you an amateur's account. These terms will come in handy later during the discussion of the lesions in specific parts of the brain.

The Central Nervous System: The brain and spinal cord, abbreviated as CNS.

The Peripheral Nervous System: Spinal nerves and cranial nerves.

The Autonomic Nervous System:

Sympathetic—Fight or flight, helps the body to deal with stress.

Parasympathetic—Controls what goes on automatically; takes care of what we are not aware of, like the heart beating.

All is controlled by the **brain** and the nerve cells, the **neurons**. The neurons have a cell body with nucleus and extensions ranging in width from sewing-thread thin to little-finger wide. These extensions are called **axons**, and they have branches called **dendrites**. (Yes, the whole network looks somewhat like a tree in winter.)

These particulars are the links that allow the neurons to communicate with each other. The neurons pick up the wish from the living person, send the commands of what to do or not to do via the axons to the dendrites. Add to that the firing of the electrical system and the release of a chemical, which help the signals from the brain to jump from one narrow gap—called a **synapse**—to another.

In more detail:

Axon: The commands from the brain travel along these strands; with the aid of chemicals, they jump from one synapse to the other to move the appropriate muscles. If the path is blocked by MS scars, the signals from the brain don't reach the muscles, the signal is distorted, or it takes too long to get from here (the brain) to there (the destination).

Dendrites: They branch off from the axons, reach toward other axons and generally are another aid in speeding up the communication process from brain to body destination.

Synapse: They are little indentations in the axon to allow the dendrites, with the aid of electro-chemicals, to assist with the brain-body communication

Brain Division: One theory holds that the brain is divided into forebrain, midbrain and hindbrain. Others call it brainstem, cerebellum and neocortex. (That is the premise I prefer.) A third one speaks of reptilian, mammalian and neocortex.

The Brainstem: It shuttles messages and impulses back and forth between the brain and the body; controls consciousness, the sleep-wake cycle, mental concentration and alertness, direction of attention and introspection. **(Please check the accuracy of this information.)** In other words, it performs one heck of a duty for the little thing it is. The cranial nerves coordinate visual activities (like reading) or set off reflex actions (like turning toward an unexpected sound.) Also located there is the medulla oblongata; it watches over breathing, heart activity, signals to swallow, sneeze or laugh.

Cerebellum: This is attached to the rear of the brainstem and is responsible for posture maintenance, coordination, muscular activities. In short, it watches over every move we make. Half of the CNS's cells are housed in the cerebellum.

As with many things that are not fully explored, there is disagreement about the cerebellum. Author Jack Fincher, who wrote *The Brain: Mystery of Matter and Mind*, (published in 1984 by Tostar Books in the series of The Human Body) says the cerebellum is called "the lesser brain." I rather agree with P.N. August; he says in *Brain Function* (published in 1988 by Chelsea House) that he finds the cerebellum "the most fascinating part of the body."

Neocortex, also called the Cerebrum: In humans, it has evolved over the millennia to the point of our present intellectually advanced state. The basics say the neocortex consists of the right and left cerebral hemispheres, connected to each other and held together by the band of fibers called the corpus callosum. Each hemisphere half is again subdivided into four lobes, each being responsible for specific actions.

The frontal lobe, located below the forehead, is responsible for reasoning and problem solving. Behind it is the parietal lobe; it contains the sensory cortex. Behind it is the occipital lobe, which contains the visual cortex, also called Brocca's brain. The temporal lobe houses the auditory cortex. It also houses Wernicke's area, which is needed to comprehend language.

The pre-frontal cortex within the frontal lobe takes care of planning and organizing, the ethical and moral sense and, along with the limbic system, has overall control over emotions. It is also associated with learning, abstract thinking, social inhibitions and intellectual functioning. It is being said to be one giant storage shed for all sorts of information.

The limbic system has come into vogue, especially since the publication of Daniel Goleman's book *Emotional Intelligence* (published by Bantam Books in 1995). An earlier book, *The ABC's of the Human Mind: A Family Book* (published by Reader's Digest Assn. in 1990) suggests the limbic system influences and somewhat modifies our behavior. It works on and with feelings. One part holds the aggression center; the other, short-term memory; another, how and what we feel and how we express our emotions.

There is one area that intrigues me and I can't find any concrete information on. It is called the reticular activating system (RAS for short) and, as I understand it, is the big filter which decides which impulses are forwarded—allowed to pass through the RAS filter—to the rest of the brain. In December 2003, my son wanted info on the RAS. I searched I don't remember how many sites; he checked them out (took him about three hours) and came back in the living room, complaining that neither site helped him any in explaining it. Well, all I could do shrug my shoulders and say, "Join the crowd. I've been searching for that for umpty dozen years," well, at least one dozen.

Okay, this is only a very rudimentary introduction to the amazing brain's many components. If you find time to look into this subject, you can be nothing but amazed over this wonder of, I say, the universe.

MSWGMD

That's enough mind-boggling for the moment, right? Let's save a tat for later and proceed now to the final segment of this introduction.

Six mistake-filled years after my multiple sclerosis diagnosis (I did a lot of denying and lying to myself), I got busy learning as much as I could. (My neighbor across the street doesn't call me a book devourer for nothing.) After I became associated with our support group, I passed that knowledge on to the group members and other interested people. Then in 1996, I decided to share it with readers and now offer it to you. Most of my theoretical knowledge came from the following sources:

Public Libraries: As with any other subject, I started my research in the public library. The greatest asset of the eight libraries I have read out are their helpful, experienced and friendly staff. The ladies at the two branches I patronize most are particularly so. I also appreciate the interlibrary loan program for books I really would like to read but which are not on the hometown library's shelves.

Allow me to relate a little MS moment. I had typed "the local branches…" and got stuck, could not think of the right word to continue. I tried attend; it didn't click. I tried go to. Nothing. I tried prefer. Nothing. So I shut the monitor off, getting up to stretch my legs and, *boing*, frequent came to my mind, and the Thesaurus helped me out with patronize. Yep, MS does play tricks on our minds, huh. I mean, tricks even Gingko Biloba can't ease.

(P.S. to the above paragraph: I pondered the patronizing during the final edit, and it hit me; I wanted to talk about the two libraries I visit primarily.)

The National MS Society: (Called the National from now on.) People who have MS may feel that they have nobody who is interested in them, nobody they can turn to. That is incorrect. There is the National with free (800) telephone numbers, friendly and helpful assistants who answer these phones and gobs of informative literature, free for the asking. Even their magazine *Inside MS* is free for those who can't afford to pay. Their extensive website contains an unbelievable quantity of quality information. The National also sponsors research projects and sets the overall tone. It is subdivided into Chapters.

The Chapters: They, too, sponsor many programs, provide leadership training, have a loan closet with a variety of items an MS person can borrow. The Chapter of course holds primarily to the opinions of the National, and in certain areas, their and my opinions differed as to what was best for our local MS support group and MS population. I will talk about that later on.

The Local Support Group: That, in my opinion, is the place to go. Different groups of course have different programs. You will be hearing a lot about ours.

Our Chief Researcher: (CR for short, remember?) One of our group members deserves special recognition. Without her tireless help, I wouldn't have been able to amass half as much information to present. Early on, even before we met in person, she wrote me a letter; we clicked and became friends. (I don't think she'd call me a friend any longer because I don't write. I sure wish she had a computer and I could fire off an e-mail now and then.) Soon after this initial communication, I received envelopes full of pertinent, annotated newspaper clippings, magazine articles, book references and even a book which explained the immune system's workings.

The Internet: Can you ever find a wealth of helpful information there! In the search field I type "Multiple Sclerosis" and add any subject I am interested in—medications, research, symptoms, for instance—and get information which keeps me busy for hours.

I also appreciate the MS websites and their bulletin boards. For a long time, I used to visit the site *www.MSWatch.com* and found some good people to interact with on their bulletin boards. Now though I mainly go to the website of the IMSSF, the International MS Support Foundation, *www.MSNews.org*, and can only praise the moderators of the bulletin boards—one strictly MS related issues, other links point to polls, general chitchat, brain teasers, a site for caregivers and several others. Jean, the founder and director, as well as volunteers Pat and Ed and the recently deceased Carole—all MS persons themselves—have put tremendous efforts into making these bulletin boards a joy to navigate. One finds helpful advice; nasty, hurtful messages are yanked, and people feel free to ask questions, ask for prayers and vent frustrations. The forums are excellent communication sources too, though I don't have time to visit there often. Another place I haven't visited is their library. All in all, I try to visit MSNews at least once a day, and I can't tell you how often I have received help, encouragement, and had my questions answered in kind, friendly, courteous, non-patronizing ways. I highly recommend this site.

There are several other very helpful Internet sites. One I have just discovered a few days ago is located at *www.mult-sclerosis.org/wholeglossary.htm*. WebMD is another worthwhile site. I have chosen

Google as my primary search engine and use My Yahoo for regular news, sports and weather.

My Story

Now let me tell you a little bit about myself.

I was born in 1938, in Germany, lived in several locations, married my husband in 1962, and in 1966, he brought me home to Marion, Ohio, which I consider my hometown.

After several stateside assignments and two tours in Vietnam, my husband was transferred back to Germany in 1970; we stayed there till 1974, and then he received his orders for Brussels, Belgium. In 1975, he retired from the Army, and we bought our house here in Galion, Ohio. In 1982, after a rather prolonged stressful time, I was diagnosed as having multiple sclerosis. (In April 2003, my husband died suddenly and totally unexpected.)

An aside: It took me some time to realize it, but I caught myself in the habit of capitalizing "Multiple Sclerosis" while writing arthritis, cancer and diabetes with small beginning letters. When I realized that, I smiled about it and changed my habit.

Now back to my story.

Points of my life are MS-important:

During my teenage years, I lived in northern Germany.

My father had multiple sclerosis.

Galion, Ohio is an MS cluster city.

I believe stress plays a major role in the development of MS and exacerbations, even if some authorities disagree with me on that one.

During critical stages in my life, I lived in the German and American MS Belt.

Diagnosis age does not equal onset age; it is just the point where a doctor of medicine confirms the diagnosis.

My onset age was traced back to age twenty-one when I had my first case of optic neuritis—blurred and double vision. After some years of relative peace and quiet (health-wise) came on-and-off uncontrollable tremors, especially when I became upset. Next, and in between, came weakness in the left arm and stiffness in the left leg, which was diagnosed as rheumatoid arthritis.

Although arthritis and multiple sclerosis are both autoimmune diseases, the different arthritis medications my family doctor prescribed didn't help. I bet he thought I was a hygiaphrontic. (That's something like having a psychosomatic illness.)

Between 1979 and 1982, the symptoms became more severe and also attacked more frequently. I got stiffer, was unsteady on my feet, couldn't keep my balance, stumbled around and fell down. At times, when I wanted to go straight, my body led me to the left and close encounters of the third kind with walls and furniture. They survived, but my body decorations stayed for a while and smarted.

The gait problems, weakness of the left side and spasticity-tremors, as well as the intellectual dysfunctions, are steady companions to this day. They get a little better during good weather (temperatures below seventy-five degrees) and worsen when it gets hot and humid and when the barometer falls. I suspect they will be with me for life. A few other odds and ends have crept up over the years, all varying in severity from day to day, sometimes from hour to hour.

In 1982, I slammed into a window—yes, it was closed—and almost went through. That's when I decided to come clean with my family doctor. He sent me to assorted specialists to have all sorts of tests performed, which, to no surprise to me, came all back clean. Grudgingly, he finally had the receptionist make an appointment with a neurologist for a consult.

(It seems to me that doctors must hate to make the multiple sclerosis diagnosis—maybe because it renders them helpless? You know, it hurts their professional pride that the healers can't heal the chronic illness?)

Well, the neurologist, after an exam, sent me to the hospital for tests—blood work, X rays, evoked responses test, spinal tap. (The MRI wasn't around at that time; I had mine a couple of years later.) On December 15, 1982, around 7:15 p.m., he gave me the MS diagnosis and sent me on my not-so-merry way of learning to live with MS.

I was lucky, sort of, I guess. I had expected the MS diagnosis because I had recognized my symptoms as resembling the ones I had observed my father suffering from and thus was mentally prepared. Oh, I wasn't exactly swelled-head proud over my medical expertise and wouldn't have minded if the doctor would have given me the famous sentence of it all being in my head. (Well, come to think of it, that would have been the truth, wouldn't it?) But he didn't laugh or pity me out of the hospital, just sent me home with a prescription for Lioresal, Prednisone and Elavil, giving me just a few days to get ready for Christmas. Thank God my kids were old enough, they no longer expected Santa Claus to dispense toys and joys.

MSWGMD

In the beginning, I made all the major mistakes possible. I refused to talk about it. I overworked, felt sorry for myself and denounced the cruel world and the uncaring people in it who didn't realize that my body had said stop. I hadn't stopped and felt bad. Of course I didn't tell them that I felt terrible.

I hope you, especially if you are newly diagnosed, are smarter and save yourself some heart-, head- and other body-aches. I also hope you will find people like my roommate in the hospital. Whenever my doctor came in the room, she went for a walk up and down the corridor. Well, she returned after the doctor had left and asked me if I had found anything out, and I told her.

"Oh, I'm sorry," she said. "That's too bad. It's an ugly disease. My niece has it too, and she's only in her twenties. She has some things wrong with her, but she doesn't let that stop her; she does almost everything she wants to, has a full-time job, goes dancing and biking."

Thanks, Helen. I'll never forget that.

More on my tries and trials, stumblings and bumblings, falling down and getting up, flips and flops, throughout this book.

I will reiterate what I said in the Foreword, in my other fiction and non-fiction works and otherwise near-preach: I place the highest value on that powerful thing called thinking. I hope the stories I tell you about myself, our group, the group members as well as what books and other people said will help you to re-think your perspective of yourself and MS. MS does make a big difference in a person's life. I had to learn to think differently about myself and my life, recognize my mistakes and make the necessary discoveries by myself. (If asked, certain people will accuse me of being bullheaded. Well, I say, to live with MS, one has to be.)

Chapter Two
What Others Say and Said

I have heard and read that MS persons want to find out as much as they can about the disease. That was and still is true for me. Over the years I have developed five ways of learning: Reading and reasoning—that is, considering and interpreting what I read, agreeing or disagreeing with it according to my experiences, judgments and beliefs. After joining the support group and the bulletin boards, I have added observing and listening, all tied together with lots of thinking.

For this chapter, I will give you my impression about books I have read and the speakers we heard at our support group meetings. Some of these books were of no personal interest to me, and I only glanced through them because I wanted to add them to the write-ups in the newsletter because I thought our members might be interested in them.

Note: These are mainly older books, but I haven't found any that explain the basics better. Quite a few of them are still on the Barnes & Noble website.

What Books Say

Mastering Multiple Sclerosis: A Guide to Management, by John Wolf, et. al., published in 1987 by Academy Books.

He has several more books out, but I find this one addresses the basics best.

This book is so full of so much info, it is nearly impossible to summarize it without running into copyright infringement trouble. I will just quote from the Table of Contents.

Mobility—from canes to wheelchairs. Access to kitchen and bathroom. Getting in the door. Public transportation.

(After reading the section on quad canes, I had my doctor prescribe me one. I still use it when I leave the house and like the feel of it. It gives more security, due to the four prongs.)

Symptoms—all well explained—spasticity, bowel and bladder problems, depression, pain, and fatigue/exhaustion.

The next section deals sensitively with relationships—marriage, sex and sexuality, children, family in general, doctor-patient relationships.

Section four explains the nervous system, diagnosis, prognosis and research. (Some of that needs to be supplemented by updated material.)

A good glossary is included, as is an extensive index. It is a good book, but to be honest, certain sections were a bit difficult to understand.

The Multiple Sclerosis Fact Book, written by Richard Lechtenberg, published in 1988 by F.A. Davis.

He, too, has written other books.

Ladies and gentlemen, this book, in my opinion, is one of the best. In the introduction he says: "The only sure thing about MS is its unpredictability." He explains the central nervous system, says that only the nerve bundles which carry information back and forth are affected, not the nerves themselves. (My note: That should give hope that they can be remyelinated, right?)

Signs of infection and inflammation show up in people who have MS, he says. White blood cells (lymphocytes) and scavenger cells (macrophages) collect in the area where the myelin is stripped. (My conjecture: This shows up later as Myelin Basic Protein, breaking through the Blood-Brain Barrier to wreak havoc in the brain or accumulating in the spinal fluid?)

Also included in the book are excellent explanations of research going on at the time of the printing, as is a chapter on what makes symptoms worse. He cites specifically that having a cold or the flu is one aggravator, as are heat, humidity, exhaustion, even not getting enough sleep. Having other major illnesses also affects the process of the MS. In other words, he says one ought to stay as healthy as possible which means, yech, exercising and eating balanced meals.

In 1995, a second edition of this book was printed, and I got hold of it. Well, here is the summary of it: As you and anybody familiar with MS can imagine, the cause is still unknown, how and why MS starts is still a mystery, how it will progress is still unpredictable, and there still is no cure. Authors, particularly those who don't have MS themselves, know the symptoms because we MSers have told them. Mr. Lechtenberg had included an update on diagnostic tests and research findings, but basically there was not that much new material in the book.

Well, I'm afraid besides the new medications and some research findings, the basic five MS questions—what is the cause, how and why does it start, specifics about
exacerbations and remissions, how will it progress, what will cure it— are still unanswered in 2002 as well as at the end of 2003 and the middle of 2004.

Symptom Management in Multiple Sclerosis, written by Randall T. Shapiro, published in 1987 by Demos Publ.

Mr. Shapiro says something can be done about MS; what that something is, he explains, comes from a program developed by the Fairview Multiple Sclerosis Center in Minneapolis.

He begins his book with a short, concise description of the brain, the nervous system and possible causes for the development of MS. Among other things, he believes in susceptibility, which appears to be at least in part genetic. MS is not inherited, he states, but a hereditary factor makes the person more susceptible to develop the disease.

He includes over-fatigue as another cause for exacerbations and provides an excellent outline of spasticity, which areas are most often affected by MS, and which exercises and specific drugs (he names them by name) will relieve symptoms.

He also describes tremors and the four types of fatigue, especially the MS fatigue, and has not forgotten to mention walking, foot drop and how to use a cane properly.

He also included wise words on proper ways to exercise, talked about diet and nutrition, vision, dizziness, vertigo, weight gain, numbness, cold feet and swollen ankles. Adapting to MS—the final chapter—gives sensible advice.

I just have to repeat myself with this one: This is one heck of a great book. I got a lot out of it and strongly recommend it. Yes, even in 2003.

P.S. Dr. Shapiro is also a volunteer consultant at the International MS Support Foundation's bulletin boards.

Multiple Sclerosis: New Hope and Practical Advice for People with MS and their Families, written by Louis Rosner and Shelley Ross, published in 1987 by Prentice Hall.

(Our CR told me a second edition had been printed, but she could not find much new material in it. I trust her judgment and haven't read it.)

I will whet your appetite with the following short description of what all is contained in this excellent book.

The authors trace the history of MS from the 1830s to the present. It contains a good description of myelin, what it does and how one's health is affected when it breaks down. In this book, I have read the first affirmation that the body can heal itself, that the plagued areas can be remyelinated. (Major, aggressive and promising research is going on in this area since 2000 and continues into the present.)

The authors detail one aspect being worked on: The human leukocyte antigen (HLA), which has a connection with the immune system, has been found in MS persons. "Maybe," they say; "a virus starts the MS and the autoimmune process keeps it going."

My note: Pretty sensible, isn't it? But I still believe the area of genetics will enter into the discussion as well as the Factor X trigger, which has yet to be discovered.

Another chapter deals with symptoms caused by lesions in specific brain areas. (I will give you my explanations about that in more detail shortly.) Also addressed: The types of MS and their prognosis, as well as a chapter talking about the causes of exacerbations.

A great piece, titled "Who handles MS best" ends this excellent book.

I had planned to do a detailed review of the above-mentioned three books and only highlight the other ones, but there is one more I found quite intriguing.

Living with Multiple Sclerosis, written by Elizabeth Forsythe, published in 1979 by Faber and Faber.

The author, an MS person herself, (I believe I remember she is a nurse) tells her story—so well known to all of us—of exacerbation and remission, the shock of the diagnosis and finding out on herself what MS is and what it does to a person. She follows that up with a chapter on the basics, but the rest is different.

She confirms my suspicions by saying that doctors are uncomfortable with diagnosing MS or dealing with a patient who has an illness they don't know much about or can't cure and follows that up with describing boo-boos inflicted by doctors on their patients.

Next comes a discussion of myths patients hang on to, what expectations they have of their neurologist and stresses the importance of acceptance. She suggests lifestyle adjustments, to adapt to the MS, but not to the point of doing less than one is capable of.

The next chapter deals with diet, nutrition, exercise and rest.

(I do have to vent my exasperation. I say "darn those people." I never liked exercising, don't have time for too much rest and can't sleep that well any longer. But her chapter called "Friends and Help" is even worse. From age sixteen on till I got married at twenty-four and again since my husband's death, I have lived alone, been responsible for myself and always hated to ask for or accept help. During my thirteen years as an Army wife, I was quite often alone with my kids while my husband was on temporary duty or while serving in Vietnam. But I never learned how to drive; now that I can't walk that much any longer, I have to rely on others to chauffeur me around, and that's tough. Ms. Forsythe, though, uses some pretty strong language, condemning those of us who don't accept help for doing things we can't do any longer and shouldn't do.)

This book also contains a good chapter on exacerbations, how to spot and prevent behavior which one knows will have a detrimental effect on one's health—exhaustion, stress, over-heating, being bothered by emotional problems. (I add "excessive worrying" to her list.)

The final chapters are as helpful.

This is a lengthy report on a paperback of 140 pages, but it is a great book. One can sense that she speaks from experience. Although it is quite old, it is still relevant. Our group's treasurer read it too, and she told me it taught her and helped her a lot.

Now a few words about books you might find interesting, beginning with three books about diets.

Multiple Sclerosis: A Self-help Guide to its Management, written by Judy Graham, published in 1984 by Thorston Publishers.

She claims MS persons suffer from certain food allergies and suggests one follow the array of recipes included in her book.

The Multiple Sclerosis Diet Book: a Low-fat Diet for the Treatment of MS, written by Ray L. Swank, published in 1987 by Doubleday.

He claims people who consume large quantities of animal fats are more prone to develop MS and offers his diet.

The Yeast Connection, written by William G. Crook, published in 1983 by Professional Books.

He talks about the relationship between Candida Albium and physical illness and describes his diet suggestions. (I have noticed newer books on this subject on the Barnes and Noble book list.)

The next two books address the concerns of the MS person's family members:

Mainstay: For the Well Spouse of the Chronically Ill, written by Maggie Strong, published in 1988 by Little Brown & Co.

The last paragraph of the Introduction says: "Mainstay is not about dying; it's about the living spouse, married to someone who is sick...through years of illness without a cure."

A sensitively written book about Mrs. Strong's coping with her husband's MS. Interspersed between her personal recollections are stories of other people and how they cope with their loved one's chronic illnesses.

Meeting the Challenge of Disability and Chronic Illness: A Family Guide, written by Lori Goldfarb, published in 1986 by Paul H. Brooks.

Many case studies show families in action. Also included are thirty-seven exercises.

I must confess, I don't particularly care for books with extensive case histories. I prefer straightforward theory, which allows me to think about what I read and form my own opinions.

The next few books don't deal directly with MS but are of interest to people with MS. The first one deals with stress.

Breaking the Stress Habit, written by Andrew Golinski, published in 1988 by Carolina Press.

The author says diet, heredity, lifestyle and environment were the causes of illness in the past, but nowadays the main health culprit is stress. (You remember, I strongly believe stress influences MS.) I believe we MSers can benefit from his advice to change and improve our attitude. Through that change, we can give our immune system some relief and let it do the work it is supposed to do—namely protect our bodies from illness instead of attacking us.

Another older book I like and still consult is *Biotypes: The Critical Link Between Your Personality and Your Health*, written by Joan Areheart-Trichel, published in 1980 by Time Books.

I haven't found another book like it nor a better one. She defines cancer, heart attack, rheumatoid arthritis and mental disorder biotypes. On the introduction's page four, she says that in times of stress, certain personality types break down and the person may develop certain illnesses. Quoting her, "In fact, certain biotypes are emerging…for diseases and disorders…that one would not suspect of having a psychological base," and mentions multiple sclerosis as one of them.

The Human Immune System: The New Frontier in Medicine, written by Steven B. Mizel, MD and Peter Jaret, published in 1986 by Simon & Schuster.

This book explains the basics of the workings of the immune system as no other one I have plowed through. The authors use language that a non-scientist can understand and can get an idea what a convoluted, complex, complicated approach the immune system uses—in the vein of, if this doesn't work, I'll try that one, and if you rascals still escape me, ha, I still have more weapons in my arsenal.

Our CR had sent me that book years ago, but it sat on my bookshelf until I decided to do this upgrade. I told my husband how great it was, and he cautioned me that many advances had been made in the meantime. I agree with that, but I maintain that the basic phraseology still is valid, and although research methods have been technically refined, the finding this book propounds are building blocks for further discoveries.

The following book needs a preamble.

In mid-1990, I had read out our local library of my kinds of books— psychology, mental health and mental illness, astrology, reincarnation, writing fiction and non-fiction books—and nobody had time to drive me to an out-of-town library. But the newsletter was due, and I wanted to include some sort of a book report.

Well, on the check-out counter lay Bernie Siegel's *Peace, Love and Healing*, and I thought that maybe some of my newsletter readers would be interested in reading a review of the subject. Maybe they had more faith in this—what shall I call it—mind over matter strong belief, faith, being able to visualize—I don't know, don't even know how to properly describe this area. Do use your own imagination and fill in my prattling with sentences which make sense.

What I wanted to say is, I branched out into the new field of that gray area with the Bernie Siegel book *Peace, Love and Healing,* written in 1990 and published by HarperCollins. (Mr. Siegel has also written another good book, titled *Love, Medicine and Miracles.*)

Up till then, I had forgotten the established fact that mind and attitude exert great influence on our psychological and physiological health. And that from me, who harps on that subject, nags at people to think, to keep a positive attitude and to never give up.

Okay, enough self-flagellation.

Mr. Siegel says when we're in the dumps, are unhappy and depressed, we feel worse than when we look at the world in a happier frame of mind, when we see how beautiful, challenging and pleasurable the world around us is.

He talks about self-induced healing—the placebo effect—which, he says, is the work of the endorphins. He adds that hope of obtaining relief, of getting well, or at least hoping to get better, has the potential of doing the healing work.

Anger has its place, he asserts. Anger held in leads to resentment and hatred. When anger is expressed, it loses its power. (I would like to add here: Anger can be expressed politely, that is, without blowing one's stack and hurting the other's feelings.)

Mr. Siegel also echoes other authors and says stress affects the immune system and may be a factor in MS and other autoimmune diseases in which the body attacks itself (Told you so, didn't I?)

He asks some thought-provoking questions: What happened a year or two before we got sick? Has any traumatic incident occurred in our life? What does the body tell us when we get sick? (See biotypes.)

And it gets worse!

Why, he asks, do we need the illness? Do we reap benefits from it?

Pages 162 to 164 are great. They talk about the survivor personality. On page 165 are lists of "How we get sick" and "How we get well."

Okay, some of my thoughts. Several times I had an insight or idea and got it confirmed by the author stating the same thought. I wrote this note in the margin: "I don't know how I should feel when other authors say the same thing I've thought before I read it. Should I be proud, glad that my thoughts are being confirmed by great or greater minds, or does it take some of the value away from my original thought?" I must confess, I swing from choice one to choice two, and sometimes come up with even choice three.

After the self-induced healing portion, I wrote in the margin: "Does he imply that our exacerbations are also self-induced?"

After the hope of relief section I wrote: "Well, I take my Lioresal and expect it to take care of the spasticity. I go on the Prednisone regime, and because it has helped me in the past, I expect it to take care of the exacerbation in the present. But I also have to consider what somebody told me: You don't know if it's the medication which made you feel better or if it's a natural remission, fabricated by your own body. I suppose I'll never know."

End of the Siegel notes. I just want to say that I did donate that book to the support group's library.

Okay, I have matured enough over my sixty-six years of living to admit to faulty reasoning. These books by authors like Siegel, as well as Borysenko and Cousin, are good reading. Reading them is no waste of time, and people who believe in these theories (no, I still don't know what I should call this area) are not pitiable dummies who have their heads in the clouds and deserve to be looked down upon. It is I who needs to be chastised for thinking myself better than others.

MSWGMD

Another book worth reading (suggested by one of our support group's speakers) is Norman Cousin's *Head First*, published in 1989 by E. P. Dutton.

It, too, makes for good, inspiring and thought-provoking reading. For those of us who prefer facts, the book includes specific background data; he names the authorities he cites and describes their research programs. He specifically outlines the essentials of a new field, that of psychoneuroimmunology (psycho: mind; neuro: brain; immunology: immune system).

This field investigates how emotions affect the body and how attitudes can help to combat serious illness. If we can make ourselves sicker, why can't we make ourselves well? he asks.

He finds the will to live of greatest importance and says that words can be lethal. (I'd say words can be more lethal than the illness when they cause the patient to give up.)

I have also looked through Joan Borysenko's book *Guilt Is the Teacher, Love Is the Lesson*, published in 1990 by Warner Books. Right at page eleven she makes the stress is bad for MS connection too.

MSWGMD

Over the years I had heard a lot about endorphins. Finally I found a book, titled *Endorphins*, written by Joel Davis, published in 1984.

Mr. Davis started the book by talking in detail about the wonder of the brain with its billions of neurons. His brain description and explanation of its workings is one of the best I have ever read—and believe me, I have read a few of them.

Endorphins are chemicals, "which make us who and what we are," he said. Their composition is similar to but hundreds of times more powerful than heroin. They are manufactured in the body without outside help. As neurotransmitters, they transfer info
between neurons and link the billions of the brain's neurons with the rest of the body.
It took a while, the researchers needed to overcome several setbacks and detours, but they found that endorphins are hormones, produced in the pituitary gland, and respond to the opiate receptors in the body. Eventually they discovered the pain-killing ability of endorphins. That is, endorphins can block release of Substance P, which initiates the response of the body to something that is painful. In plain language, it says that an increase in endorphins can relieve pain. But the more

exciting news is that they influence the immune system for the better and we ourselves can stimulate the production of more endorphins, which can lead to a feeling of greater well being.

In 1975, a research team found out, and it has been verified in other studies many times, that the body produces endorphins in response to stressful situations. You have probably heard the reports about runner's high, that runners are getting a second wind to finish the race after they had thought they were ready to fall down on the spot from sheer exhaustion.

Know what scientists found in the bodies of these runners? Yep, a giant amount of endorphins. This proves that exercising increases the level of endorphins. (Thank goodness the computer can't transpose a tongue stuck out at it.) I don't remember if it was in the Norman Cousin or the Bernie Siegel book (mentioned earlier), but I remember that in either of those two it was mentioned that a good belly laugh also increases the production of endorphins. Our treasurer, who liked to laugh, also caught on to that.

Three experiments in 1982 confirmed that endorphins influence the immune system. (Did your ears just perk up as mine did when I read that?) It is being said that injection of enkephalin or endorphins helps the T-cells. Also, arthritis sufferers have decreased amounts of endorphins in their blood. I do wonder: Has anybody checked the endorphin levels in MS persons, particularly during an exacerbation? Darn it, sometimes I wish MSers could work with scientists and point them in the right direction. As I said so many times, we are the ones who live with the disease and could provide practical, not only theoretical, knowledge. But I guess nobody asks us, huh.

Okay, back to the endorphins.

I have checked in three area libraries but can't find a newer book on endorphins. The only one on the shelves was *the Pleasure Connection: How Endorphins Affect Our Health and Happiness*, written by Deva and James Beck, published in 1987 by Synthesis Press.

It is written in less technical tones than the Davis book, with applications to everyday life, emotions and well-being. It also shows ways to stimulate production of endorphins, though I must say I wasn't too impressed with it.

Well, I did return to Old Faithful (Google Search Engine) and found some endorphin info, short and to the point, on the *www.biotech-usa.com* site. It said that since 1987, endorphin research has advanced considerably. By now, twenty different types of endorphins have been named. It is being reiterated at this site too that endorphins relieve pain, but it also said that they relieve stress symptoms. An item in the section "What are the Endorphins doing in our body?" states that they "enhance our immune system." A later list details the seven benefits of endorphins, and number six states another fact I had not been aware of: Endorphins aid in improving our memory.

That ends the book list. As I have mentioned earlier, the National has a veritable gold mine, a treasure throve of brochures, pamphlets and booklets on every imaginable subject, yours for the asking.

Chapter Three

What Doctors, Occupational Therapists, Physical Therapists and Group Members Said

The information in this section came to me via people who spoke to our group. I have also included things our group members said and wrote.

Our group's first president had arranged with a neurologist to answer written questions. It didn't last long, not being the doctor's fault; the questions trickled to a stand-still.

Here is one of those questions and answers:

Q. "Dear Doctor,

"Sometimes it seems like my MS is so different from others who have MS. Why is that so?

"The Odd One."

A. "Dear Odd One,

"MS has no set pattern; it is as individual as the person diagnosed with it. All you can do is bear with it and threat the symptoms as they come and go.

"Best of health."

Another set:

Q. "Dear Doctor,

"When I have things I feel I must get done in a certain time frame, I push myself until it is done. This sometimes means that I have exhausted myself to the point that I must rest up to seven days to recuperate. Will this affect my disease in the long run?

"Pusher."

A. "Dear Pusher,

"Exhaustion should be avoided, as it may lead to a temporary increase in other symptoms. The long-term effect is not clearly understood. If you must undertake a tiring task or one that will take a prolonged period of time, try to do it in steps with frequent rest periods before continuing. A one- or two-hour nap may help rejuvenate you. Try and plan your activities for the early morning hours when you have the most energy. Again, the key may be in recognizing your limits, that is, realizing that it may vary from day to day.

"Best of health."

MSWGMD

In the following section, I will tell you a little what guest speakers taught us. Maybe that will inspire you to invite such individuals to your support group? My updating comments are found in parentheses.

One of the first speakers was a neurologist; he spoke about the physiology of MS, showed slides of the brain, pointed out lesions and explained the process of diagnosis. (That was before the MRI became a common diagnostic tool.) He also spoke about available medications—Lioresal for spasticity; Symmetrel, an anti-viral drug, aiding in smoother conduction of nerve signals; Tegretol for face pain. Of course today a neurologist would talk about the ABCRs, Solu-medrol, neurontin, provigil and others. He also spoke of copolymer-1 (cop-1, as we used to call it, which was already used in Israel) and mentioned that it should become available within months. (Ha! Later on I'll tell you the story of cop-1's thorny path leading to Copaxone's approval by the FDA.)

MSWGMD

Lots of info got packed into another meeting. A nurse from an area hospital spoke about "Energy conservation," and outlined briefly what the hospital had to offer. I have incorporated a few of her excellent and timely hints and suggestions in my daily routine. For instance, she suggested to rearrange your house/work area to decrease steps and get more done with less overexertion.

Plan ahead but be flexible. Don't worry about things you can't do anything about and can't change.

Don't push yourself, work during your peak hours, take rest periods and relax.

Next a representative of a wheelchair company explained the wheelchair he had on display. He gave tips and hints on how to choose a wheelchair and what to look for. "Ask the salesperson questions," he advised. "Make sure you choose one that fits your specific needs and serves your purpose." An MS person who uses the wheelchair outside needs one with different wheels than if it is used strictly in the house.

"Lastly," he said, "be sure to buy quality from someone knowledgeable, look for the warrantee and sit in it long enough to ensure that it is comfortable."

The natives got restless, that is, we were getting stiffish and our chairperson called for the seventh inning stretch. After that, a representative of a hearing aid company took the floor. She showed slides prepared by the Better Hearing Institute and spoke about hearing impairments, what and how the doctor tests, which types of hearing aids are available and what one can expect after being fitted with one.

MSWGMD

Another time an ophthalmologist spoke on "MS and the Eye." He defined MS as a "disseminating disease, demyelinating the white matter of the brain." Turning to specific eye problems, he spoke in detail about different phases and problems of optic neuritis.

Optic neuritis, he said, is an inflammation of the optic nerve; the symptoms include blurred, cloudy and double vision. The frequency of optic neuritis attacks determines if permanent vision damage will occur because with each attack some nerve fibers die. He also said that the inflammation suggests a viral link.

Cortico steroids (prednisone), taken on a short-term basis, often help MS patients, he said. (I can attest to the fact that it does so.) He stressed that much research was going on but that much more was needed.

By now it is understood that optic neuritis is an almost-sure sign of MS. As I mentioned before, my ophthalmologist had confirmed that.

MSWGMD

During one of our meetings, our president had us consider the five steps most people diagnosed with multiple sclerosis go through. She called them "Denial, Anger, Bargaining, Depression and Acceptance." After handing out pencils and paper, she asked us to write down how we related to that and had us read our answers out loud.

(That was the first time I was able to speak up and am I ever glad I did. How I reached that point, I'll explain later.)

After the first go-around, she asked the MSers in the group to share how we coped. Two sets of points crystallized:

1. MS persons, as a group, are one darn strong bunch of people.

2. The support of family and friends is very much appreciated.

Here is an interesting point though. One time we had a divided meeting where people with MS talked in one room and the caregivers—family and friends—talked about their concerns in another. At that meeting we strictly talked about ourselves and our difficulties of coping with MS. But you know what? I have never found out what the caregivers said, darn them. (Of course I tried to find out. Only to, *ahem*, make life easier for them by changing what they disliked. Do you believe me? No? Now my feelings are hurt.)

MSWGMD

During another meeting, we again had three speakers, with all three providing excellent insights and information.

Speaker number one was an occupational therapist from a rehab center. She explained her mission as "trying to help people with disabilities to help themselves to be productive members of society."

She showed gadgets that assist in independent living, help conserve energy or items which were simply useful—reachers, bathtub benches and toilet seat raisers, bath mittens, aids to close buttons and zippers, build-up eating utensils, canes and walkers. These items can be obtained through pharmacies, rehab centers or departments of hospitals. Many insurance companies pay for them if a doctor writes a prescription.

She also explained how rehab centers can aid a person through their Independent Living Programs; they can provide equipment, do home adaptations, build outside ramps for easier access, or, sometimes with the help of a state's Bureau of Vocational Rehabilitation, they even install stair lifts.

A physical therapist spoke next. She said their goal is "attaining the highest possible level of independent living" and stressed the importance of family involvement in the rehab and therapy process. "The family must be informed," she said.

A dietician spoke about nutrition, the need for balanced meals and keeping adequate rest periods. She also said MS persons have to have at least three hours of fun a day. Not to forget the necessity for regular exercise, it helps relieve stress. (The endorphins, remember?)

MSWGMD

After three cancellations due to bad Ohio winter weather, the third time was a charm, and we heard a nurse speak on the subject of "Humor, Laughter and Healing." This lady had crippling rheumatoid arthritis and was somewhat handicapped herself; thus, some of her suggestions and advice evolved through personal experience.

She started out comparing arthritis and MS—both are autoimmune diseases; both are, at present (2004), incurable; both are associated with the failings of the immune system. Both also put the sufferer on an emotional rollercoaster. In fact, she said, while preparing herself for this talk, she had marveled how much alike arthritis and MS appear to be.

To cope, a good sense of humor is a must, she asserted, and so is the ability to see the humor in ordinary things if one expects to survive living with a chronic, debilitating disease. That does not mean one makes fun of a person or the illness; it's just that humor helps. When we grin at it, it becomes much easier to bear the burden which life heaps on us. Humor lifts the spirit, decreases depression, and a good belly laugh takes away the pain. (Because it increases the endorphins and blocks release of Substance P, remember?)

So, she advised, focus on the positive and laugh. Talk to yourself and tell yourself something nice. Give yourself a boost and do the same for somebody who may be depressed.

Another uplifting evening with lots to think about.

MSWGMD

The mother of a young man who had chronic-progressive MS and died believed strongly that heavy metals, mercury and lead in particular, play a role in Galion's preponderance of MS cases. (My Factor X being an environmental trigger, I heard that being mentioned.) Mrs. H. has assembled a veritable library of material supporting her theory and presented some highlights to our group. She gave a detailed overview of the field and bolstered her theory with written and video proof.

Our chairperson picked up and ran with that ball, prepared and gave a detailed report. The following segment is based on that talk.

She began with discussing dentist Hal Huggins' book *It's All in the Head*. (I'm sorry, I can't find publication data.)

Dr. Huggins points out that an amalgam filling is composed of fifty percent mercury and mercury is considered to be highly toxic, giving off measurable vapors and that, he asserts, is highly detrimental to a person's health. The poison does not actually cause the MS, but it mimics many illnesses and causes exacerbations. According to the book, many MS patients who had their amalgam fillings replaced with composite ones saw improvements, in some cases, dramatic ones.

But, Dr. Huggins said, these are facts that most doctors of medicine or dentistry refuse to discuss, acknowledge or give credence to.

Next we watched two videos on this subject. In the first, more general one, several patients described their symptoms, physicians, dentists and nutritionists gave their view (factual pros and cons), and several of the narrators kept referring to mercury's effects on the immune system.

Video number two was Louise Herbeck's story of *How I Conquered Multiple Sclerosis*. She is a diagnosed MS patient and described in detail how she had suffered with severe MS symptoms and had completely recovered after her amalgam fillings had been removed and replaced. (I don't remember if she was in permanent remission or found to be MS-free.)

For the next two meetings, our chairperson picked up that skein of wool and ran with it. She shared the list of potential physical, physiological, mental or emotional troubles which, according to the critics of amalgam fillings, could beset a person with these fillings: Psychological disturbances, oral cavity disorders, effects on the gastrointestinal area, neurological, cardiovascular, respiratory, immunological and endocrine problems. She also had unearthed a report of "The Foundation for Toxic-free Dentistry." Their members believe that mercury should not be placed in people's mouths, and if any symptoms of mercury poisoning are present, steps should be taken to remove the mercury from teeth and body.

To be fair, she also requested a statement from the National as to their position of this subject. Their conclusions are paraphrased, not verbatim:

1. There are no indications that a higher incidence of MS exists among dentists or oral assistants.

2. There is a seventy percent placebo effect in MS patients, which makes it difficult to evaluate improvements. A consensus among physicians is to avoid unnecessary surgery or anesthesia.

3. It involves economic implications.

4. If the person was helped, maybe they were misdiagnosed.

5. There is no bonafide evidence.

This concludes our chairperson's report. Now I want to put in my five cents' worth. No, considering inflation, make that fifteen.

In answer to the National's reply, I say this: Regarding number one: Do the dentists and assistants have mercury in their teeth? Regarding number five: The misdiagnosis suggestion is the pits! I would have accepted a referral to the possibility of spontaneous remission—but that, a misdiagnosis? Come on! To me, it sounds like contrived hyperbole, used as an excuse or an attempt to justify a point of view.

I have often thought, said and heard others lament the fact that the National stubbornly insists on only their beliefs always being correct. Some of the points outlined above, don't they sound so artificial and fabricated as to sound silly?

Incidentally, not many people working at the National or the Chapter have multiple sclerosis themselves. Many people, MSers and non-MSers alike, raise their eyebrows when they hear that. How can these people understand what a person who has the erratic disease of MS goes through or what is important to them? (The founder and the moderators of the IMSSF—my favorite website and bulletin boards, remember—all have multiple sclerosis.)

Anyway, the end of the group's mercury discussion was not the end of the controversy. CBS's *60 Minutes* ran a piece on this debate, leaning toward a guilty verdict—at least that was what it sounded like to me. Dan Rather, the anchor of *CBS Evening News*, also discussed it at least once during the regular half-hour evening news.

To these reports, the National issued another denunciation and stubbornly clung to their standpoint. I swear, they're as unbending as the Freudian psychoanalysts and the Catholic Church.

(I wish I could kick myself—or the guilty party—for having lost the notes of dates, times and other specifics about the above-cited CBS facts. I hope CBS forgives me. Too bad that I can't distort my body to reach my you-know-what to kick it.)

Oh, the Reader's Digest's *ABC of the Human Mind*, published in 1990 by Reader's Digest, has an interesting item. An insert on page thirty-six talks about the olden times and how hat makers suffered from muscular tremors, mental confusion, slurred speech and other such ailments. From these symptoms was coined the expression "Mad as a hatter." This behavior, it was stated in the book, was caused by the poisonous, mercury-laden vapors the workers inhaled while making felt hats.

Now the decision rests with you.

Well, not quite. I was just on the Internet, checking for the status of cladribine therapy, and what do I see on the side bar? A link to the website *www.noamalgam.com*. It describes a book, and the info states that mercury poisoning is more common than imagined. The illnesses associated with it (or caused by it) can be cured. (That was in 2002.)

MSWGMD

The following is a report on a comprehensive, all-encompassing question and answer session Dr. Rammohan conducted at our support group. I had been a patient of his and had invited him to speak to our group. Graciously he had consented to do so.

Dr. Rammohan, at that time (May 1990), was associate professor of neurology at the Ohio State University Hospitals and served as director of the Multiple Sclerosis Clinics at OSU. He is also a National MS Society grantee and over the years has contributed valuable research data.

In addition to all the above, he is also a humane physician, the one who is considered the doctor to send MS patients to when other physicians and neurologists (of course I know that neurologists are physicians; I just wanted to make the distinction between the general practitioner and the specialist) declare themselves near-defeated.

Dr. Rammohan began his presentation with a short introductory speech, talked about the viral connection, the genetic link and said it was thought that four specific genes were faulty and had been found in MS patients. (This area is still very high on the research priority list in 2004.)

He scorned the flutter of the news media about so-called cures appearing with regularity and warned of another one being in the making.

Next he gave a detailed overview of the workings of the immune system, how it is supposed to fight invaders, that it makes mistakes, losing the "recognition of self," falls apart and leaves the body open to attack. He addressed specific research going on, not only in the United States, but all over the world. He also discussed the heredity factor. MS is not inherited, he stated; just in ten percent of MS patients is there another close family member who has MS, and MS rarely, if ever, attacks more than two generations.

(Well, I disagreed then, and in 2004, I disagree even more. If you read postings on MS bulletin boards or ask the question if somebody has a relative who has MS, you will learn facts. It's tough to believe in the conclusions of some statisticians. It might also be interesting who funded these studies?)

Regarding the stress-flare-up connection, he gave a qualified no between the two. He said we happen to remember the exacerbation we had after a stressful event but forget the one we had after a happy time. But, he emphasized, it makes sense to live an as stress-free life as possible.

(Well, I call stress any too much, be that good and bad, happy and sad, emotionally uplifting and emotionally devastating and count exacerbations following either of these events.)

He spent considerable time on discussing medications. (As I warned earlier, this event, too, occurred before the appearance of the ABCRs.) He mentioned Cyclosporine. It is not a magic cure, he said, but it does slow down chronic-progressive MS. This has been established as fact because chronic-progressives get better on cyclosporin but not on their own. Symmetrel, or the generic amantadine, improves nerve impulse conduction and helps alleviate fatigue in some MS patients. (I think I said it before that it's an anti-viral and there is a virus link associated with MS.) Lioresal, or the generic baclofen, improves spasticity in some patients. Cortico steroids, prednisone, are designed for short-term use. If it is taken for too long a period, it can cause serious side effects. And never stop prednisone cold turkey; the body has to be weaned off the medication slowly.

I hesitate mentioning the next medication, because in 1996, I had been told it was no longer prescribed. I still have not verified if the new infused medication, called Solu-Medrol, belongs in the same category as ACTH was. I say this because Dr. Rammohan mentioned ACTH, (adrenocorticotropic hormones), which was administered intravenously and was said to halt an exacerbation. He also spoke of several medications that were in the development stage. (I never got an ACTH regime because a) I didn't want to lie around in the hospital, and b) because I had heard that these infusions had to be taken on an ever-increasing time span. I believe it is the same with solu-medrol.)

Other questions he provided answers to: Diagnosing MS. Thanks to the MRI, it is now possible to say firmly, "Yes, it is MS." Of course, he said, there are still cases where all the tests come back clean while everything looks as if the patient has MS. That is as frustrating for the doctor as it is for the patient.

Definitions he used: Clonus is a jerking of the limbs, occurring especially during the night. He defined spasticity as "leg stiffness," it being worst in the morning. He suggested taking one's first dose of Lioresal one or two hours before getting up.

Specific or high doses of vitamins don't really help, but if you find them of benefit, keep on taking them, but be careful. It has been established that even the water-soluble ones—the B and C vitamins—in high doses can be toxic and harm you.

(My neurologist has advised me on my very first visit to take a daily multi-vitamin, and even after over ten years as his patient, he still asks frequently if I'm taking them regularly. I also take Ginko Biloba and believe in its efficacy; if I don't take it, my speech deteriorates and becomes riddled with "uh, ah and oh." So I know it works for me.)

In regards to wheelchairs and scooters, he had this to say: Many MS patients believe the old hat of "Once you're in the wheelchair, you'll never get out of it." That's a myth, he said. Use one if necessary. They are helpful, make you less dependent on others, and you're less restricted in your movements. They also can improve your productivity, and you can join your friends and family on many outings you'd otherwise miss if you'd refuse to avail yourself to its convenience.

After a few closing remarks and generalized questions, we thanked Dr. Rammohan for coming the fifty miles and getting lost in our detour-riddled city and raided the well-stocked refreshment table. He stuck around another hour to patiently and knowledgeably answer our personal questions. I still say this doctor is one of the greatest. (Although I still wish I could clone my neurologist to make sure I have him for the rest of my life.)

A Personal Aside

1. As I said, this talk happened in 1990, but do you realize everything Dr. Rammohan said then (except for the medication field) is still up-to-date today? As I say and said so many times, not much has significantly changed over the years.

2. This is what I wrote in 1996.

How do you who are still mobile feel about the wheelchair business? I admit, I've only been able once to take that advice and that was when my husband had carotid artery surgery; I let the nurses and my daughter-in-law persuade me to use it because I wouldn't have been able to get around on my own for twelve hours, but otherwise, I said, uh-uh.

As I told my neurologist, I think it's my independent streak, my pride of being in control, of doing for myself. I'd feel sort of ashamed to depend even more on others than I already do.

If you fall in the same category, well, don't feel bad; we're allowed a few quirks, foibles and idiosyncrasies.

Or could it be that despite all my erudite words I still, *ahem*, haven't completely accepted that I, *uh*, have multiple sclerosis?

About five years ago (May 1999), I changed my outlook. My son-in-law, as a birthday present, gave me a ticket to attend a Reds baseball game in Cincinnati, Ohio. People who had been at the stadium before warned me of the long walk from the parking lot to the area where our seats were located. Well, I did do the walking on the way in, and wow, did I pay for it. But after the game, Matt nabbed one of the security guards, requested a wheelchair, and the guard wheeled me to the car.

The year after that, I received another ticket, but this time we packed my wheelchair in the trunk, and Matt gave me a ride. I could enjoy the game unexhausted and didn't have to recuperate for a week after the game.

I won't say that I wasn't a bit uncomfortable—actually a little ashamed—for being unable to transport myself from point A to point B, but if I get another ticket to a game by the Reds, Indians, Browns, Bengals or OSU football, I'll climb in the wheelchair again.

Last May, my daughter and some friends invited me to attend a retreat with them. I knew there would be a lot of walking. I called the cabin, reserved a wheelchair and enjoyed the thirty-six hours without total exhaustion.

So, that's me, and another one of my mind changes. As I said above, how do you feel about this wheelchair business?

Now back to what others said.

MSWGMD

During another meeting, two self-defense specialists addressed our group. The two ladies, one not much taller than five-foot-two and a size eight, the other taller and more compact, sure knew their subject and presented some darn good suggestions.

They began with a detailed report on sexual assaults, which can happen to both women and men, they said, and then provided information on how to respond and defend oneself.

Prevention is the best and easiest thing to do. If you are the victim of a sexual assault or other violent crime, go to the hospital and be examined and also report it to the police. Reporting it does not mean it has to be prosecuted; it just means making the police aware of what is going on in the community.

Many people are unaware that most states have victim's compensation programs and only three percent of people eligible for this compensation apply for it.

Begin your self-defense program by thinking about what to do if it should happen. Don't say, "It won't happen to me"; it might, so be prepared. Realize that men are stronger from the waist up and women are stronger from the waist down. If you plan to use a key to defend yourself, use only one and aim for the eye.

Additionally, they said: Be alert. Pay attention to your surroundings and what goes on around you. There is strength in numbers—use the buddy system. Keep a knife or open pocketknife handy; also keep one under the mattress.

Over and over, both ladies stressed: Be aware. Lock the doors when you are alone. It's better to appear a little paranoid—overly cautious— than getting hurt. Don't let strangers into your house unless they properly identify themselves, especially not when you are alone with small children. Robbers, rapists and other criminals may threaten to hurt your kids to force you to do their bidding, so don't advertise that you have kids by leaving toys and bikes lying openly in the front yard.

If you are in a wheelchair, put your purse—preferably a clutch purse or pencil case—behind your back. The disability already works against a person, makes them easier prey, so be extra careful. Don't make it easier for them.

Mace is not really effective; it gives a false sense of security, the speaker said, and proved her point by asking a 5'4" MS woman and a 6' man to demonstrate. She didn't have much of a chance against the man who could move much quicker than the slower-moving and more-unsteady-on-her-feet handicapped woman. Before she had the pretend-mace bottle chest high and was ready to extend her hand, he had already reached her, pretended to slap it out of her hand and immobilized her.

Summary: Be prepared. Be alert. Be aware of what is going on around you.

I related how my mother had insisted I carry some black pepper in my jacket or coat pocket when I had to be out after dark. While working in a drug and alcohol assistance center and the director and the counselors all had to leave, my supervisor insisted I had a pair of scissors next to my right hand. Later on, while my husband was on his tours of duty in Vietnam, I was alone with two young boys, and at his second tour of duty, with the boys and a baby girl. I used the scissors defense preparation and also kept a baseball bat near both front and back doors.

I still keep one bat by the back door and one in the living room to threaten my sometimes-not-so-beloved family members when they, uh, don't act so lovingly. I also offer said device's use as well as the iron skillet to my son-in-law and daughters-in-law.

MSWGMD

A while ago I talked with my neurologist about my observation that I'm quite unsteady when I walk looking up or straight ahead and that I have more control when I look down on my feet and watch them. Walking just a few steps in the dark is gruesomely scary. (That's why my son-in-law bought, and my husband installed, a security light by the backdoor which lights up when a person or car approaches the ramp.)

The doctor asked me why I thought that was so, and I replied with the cerebellum-brainstem reference. He had a better explanation, easier to follow too, because I understood what was going on and am not completely at my body's mercy.

We need four functions when we walk, he explained. The feet touch the ground and evaluate it—is it even, steep, rocky? The eyes observe, particularly a step or two ahead. The brain directs the muscles to move. The muscles move the feet.

Since in some MS persons, one, two or even three of these senses are impaired, we have to compensate. Of course we are less secure on our feet and must watch each step more closely, not to forget that maybe the brain-muscle or brain-feet nerves may be damaged so we need the eyes to counterbalance.

And he told me that way before it came out in a research paper from the National, which to me, proves he is keeping on top of new research. No wonder I am comfortable with him.

I also wish to stress once again that these suggestions were offered between 1988 and 1993, but they are still as relevant today (November 2003) as they were then.

Wise Words from Our Group Members

Our chairperson contributed the following: (I add: I believe these suggestions could be used year-round, especially by housebound MSers.)

Welcome to December. I suppose I'm not the only one with the winter/holiday blues. I have read several newspaper articles about stress and depression around the holidays. They suggest reducing it and doing things you enjoy, not sticking to tradition if it causes more stress than enjoyment. So start your own holiday traditions.

I have already started to get "house-claustrophobia" from the icy weather and being down with a cold. I suggest finding something you enjoy doing and pass the winter safely. I spent an entire morning cleaning neglected blinds, woodwork and cobwebs. Surprisingly, I felt much better afterwards. [All I say to that is yech and double yech.]

Jigsaw puzzles, reading books, doing needlework, playing my clarinet and listening to my favorite music are some things I plan for lonely days in winter. I think that by planning ahead and stocking up I will be better able to fight off the winter blues.

Also, I suggest getting out when it is a clear, sunny day. You can't count on it to last long, so force yourself to get out. Exercising, too, can keep you moving even if you are inside. [Triple yech.] Burning a scented candle helps freshen the air in the house. Try it.

Remember, too, if depression gets you down and you can't shake it, contact your physician; there are medications that can help.

She has also written the following:

Forces of the Unknown (Multiple Sclerosis)

MS forced me to change my life.

I was a full-time radiologist in the diagnostic radiology and computerized technology (CAT Scan) department of a mid-sized community hospital. I had two children—then ages one and four. I worked two to ten hours of overtime a week and was "on call" up to sixty hours a week. My husband worked part-time evenings and watched our kids during the day. I loved my job but also felt guilty about the lack of time with my family.

After five years, my disease forced me to realize that I could no longer do my job at the hospital. It took time to adjust to the changes and depression came occasionally, but having MS also added positive forces to my life.

It forced me to slow down and appreciate my surroundings.

It forced me to face my physical limitations.

It forced me to become closer to my husband.

It forced me to stop and notice my two wonderful, energetic, creative young boys.

It forced me to pay more attention to living a healthy lifestyle.

It forced me to look inside myself.

And what's so bad about that?

MSWGMD

Our treasurer wrote the following poem:

Life

I had lost all joy and hope. My heart was filled with a very heavy load.

I walked out in the sunlight to breathe clean, fresh air.

I walked a mile or two and asked myself: Why feel so blue?

I looked around and saw that there were daffodils blooming and the grass was green and a blue sky all around.
Then clouds began to form.
The rain fell gently to the ground and I walked on back toward home.
I told myself: The clouds must come. The rain must fall.
If not, there would be no daffodils or crops to grow.
So this is life to live at your best. We must accept, no matter what we do.
Clouds will disappear and the sun will shine again.
Our love and joy sets hearts aglow with life's ambitious glory.

She also wrote the following:

Courage
Courage is someone who never gives up. You never want to say you can't do it.
You might stumble and fall but you must pick yourself up and try again and again.
Just remember one thing: There is only one you and you are important.
God never gives you more than you can handle.

MSWGMD

Our first chairperson wrote the following:

I Can't Stand It!
   Have you ever reached the point where the thoughts and physical limitations of multiple sclerosis led you to believe you couldn't stand it for another minute? The point at which you felt as if it was hopeless to continue to live a life that is totally unfair and worthless?

When you feel this way, you need to be realistic with yourself and remind yourself of a few facts.

1. No matter what you do, say or think, you can't change the fact you have MS.

2. There are no cures or answers to rule out symptoms and paralysis that accompany multiple sclerosis.

3. You have no choice but to accept and deal with the life you now lead.

Also, remind yourself that you are a strong person and convince yourself that you can handle anything that life deals up. If all else fails, be glad it is you who has MS rather than anyone you love.

MSWGMD

I commiserated with a group member about fatigue, how tough it is to deal with and how difficult a task it is to make non-MSers understand it. I added: "And I feel so guilty when I see all the work that waits for me and here I hang in my chair, unable to keep my eyes open and do something."

Had I been fatigued at that moment, her answer surely would have jarred me awake. "Why feel guilty?" she asked. "Work doesn't fly away; it'll be here when you get around to it. Relax and wait till you feel better, and you'll feel better faster if you don't fuss."

You know something? Of course she was right. I now try to relax as long as nobody's life, limb, emotional or physical health is jeopardized. Or, right now I add, as long as my four-year-old grandson doesn't alert me with being too quiet.

One more wise saying:

On assuming her office, our last chairperson started her first meeting as the new group leader with offering the following three sentences for consideration and discussion.

1. Share your smile.
2. Nobody is so poor that they can't give.
3. Nobody is so rich that they can't take.

Good piece as food for thought, isn't it.

MSWGMD

I debated where to offer the following two inspirational presentations—put it among the discussion about what speakers said or place it in the "Encouragments" section? Well, I decided to offer them as endings to this chapter.

A counselor from the Rehab Services of North Central Ohio Inc. dealt with the subject of Stress and Frustration in Dealing with Ms. I found it inspiring just to look at him, a young man, handicapped himself, coping matter-of-factly and admirably with his disability. I called him a few days later at work, conveyed my congratulation and requested reprint permission of the handout he had provided. He gave me permission, and here is it.

Dealing with Stress and Frustration:

1. Analyze the situation—is there pressure? Is it from yourself? Others?
2. What is the desired goal? What is the actual achievement? How different are they? [He had amended that with: What do you want to achieve? What results or rewards will you receive? Is it worth the effort?]
3. What message are we or others sending?
4. How valid is the message? [Belief?]

Beliefs/Messages: [we send ourselves which cause frustration and stress]

She'll be angry/upset, won't understand. I'll feel guilty, will blame me.
It will be my fault; they'll think I'm stupid, lazy, ignorant, insensitive.
She'll kill me. They won't like me any more. They'll be really disappointed in me.
I'll feel rejected. I'll be fired. I won't be loved.

Techniques: [to relieve the stress and frustration]

Talk it over with a neutral person.
Review similar experiences, check if your messages are valid.
Use humor.
Adjust your values/beliefs and goals. [I'd add: toward reality.]
Get away from the situation.
"Reward" yourself for toughen it out.
Use relaxation exercises.
Seek support—support groups, counseling.
Prayer
Learn about stress and how to deal with it.
Get adequate rest and proper diet, medical care.
Adjust your performance realistically.
Discuss your beliefs with the other person involved. (Be honest about your feelings and responses.)

The above is from a talk given by Larry Bocka, SCSW, LISW Rehabilitation Services of North Central Ohio, 270 Sterkel Blvd., Mansfield, OH 44907.

MSWGMD

The speaker of the following piece is very dear to me; she is my daughter-in-law. She is a nurse, and at the time she addressed our group, she was working in an area hospital in the rehabilitation department. A while ago, she changed jobs and recently received the employee-of-the-month award. Yes, I not only love her but also am proud of her and trust her. Now she is working in a major hospital and was my Avonex trainer. I tell you, she is good.

At her presentation, she jumped right in at the meaty part. She stressed several times that we should consult our physician for a program of physical therapy or other exercises.

Two other recurring themes in her talk: 1. Have and hold a positive attitude. 2. Stay mobile.

Her definition of rehabilitation: Achieving the highest level of function—even if you need to use a cane, walker or wheelchair, use whatever means you need to achieve the maximum possible.

Exercise starts in the mind; our brain is the largest organ—keep it mobile. [Through thinking, I'd say.]

Stay as active as possible but get adequate rest. Eat a good, balanced diet. Avoid people who have a cold.

Even if you have lain flat in bed, you can get back into shape and achieve at least some sense of mobility.

When you exercise or are enrolled in a rehab program, keep at it. Don't think: It's not that bad if I'll just skip it this one day. It is that bad. But don't get discouraged either; don't give up. Positive thinking works. You don't have anything to lose but a lot to gain.

But don't deceive yourself: It will be rough. Prepare yourself with medication, according to your doctor's instructions. Work on a daily basis, seven days a week.

Even those in wheelchairs can and should exercise. It not only keeps you in shape, it also keeps you limbered up and more independent.

Set small, realistic goals; don't go for the whole block at once. Be proud when you have achieved a goal. Reward yourself, and it will be easier to convince your mind to go on to the next goal and work toward achieving it.

The more and the longer you work, the better you get. Practice does make perfect.

Use the adaptive devices; they can make your life easier, make you more productive and keep you independent.

Again she stressed to start any program with a visit to the doctor and suggested to exercise with a group of people, maybe even during the support group meeting.

When you hurt, you have done too much. Never exercise to the point of hurting. Wear your brace when you exercise. If you are unsteady and stagger, use your cane.

An interesting point: The best people to invent something are those who need it.

Ask yourself: What can I do—physically, mentally and emotionally? How can I get around the problem? Also analyze the problem.

[It would be a good idea to use the points suggested by Mr. Bocka, as outlined in the previous segment.]

Apply pressure to make things and places more handicapped-accessible.

Don't be embarrassed about being handicapped. Be courageous enough to explain that you have MS, what MS is, how it affects you and how it makes you feel. [I would add: Practice that speech so you can deliver it factually, especially if you are a bit intimidated.]

People put too many limitations on themselves. Don't concentrate on what you can't do; concentrate on what you can do. Use your imagination. Improvise. Don't push yourself too hard, or you might regress, but even the smallest achievement is important. Stay as mobile as possible. And never give up on yourself.

Those were the major points, and now you know why I'm so darn proud of my daughter-in-law.

Chapter Four
What I Have Learned

For this chapter I need to beg your indulgence. There is so much information out there and many studies and reports regarding research, theory, treatment and medications overlap. That is, many of the following individual entries fit into two or sometimes even all categories. I have tried to group the subjects together as much as possible, but it still may appear as if it were thrown together haphazardly. Please do bear with me.

Few Preparatory Words

I have often expressed in written and spoken words my certitude of scientists coming ever closer to discovering what causes MS, what provokes exacerbations, what brings on remissions. Well, in mid-1991, I figured it had become time to back my verbal words with documentation. I'll admit that I didn't do it only for the group members but also for myself, to steady myself on. It doesn't happen very often, and I confess it rarely, but sometimes I do slither into the dumps of doubts too, am convinced that nothing will ever change except that it will get worse. Thus putting this report together provided some hope and healing relief for me, too.

Of course seeing the wealth of information accumulated in the intervening twelve years spurned me on even further to do these updates. Thus this chapter includes both old and newer material.

MSWGMD

My kids used to call me a psychology nut and book worm. (They also insisted that I'm a ring and watch freak and a pen thief; I plead guilty to all four.) It's true, I love to read and learn new things, but for the longest time, I had no interest in studying the brain and thought even less about investigating the field of genes. (Maybe my mind was scared of the magnitude of the two fields and how the learning process would never stop.)

Well, finally the neuro in neuromuscular got to me; I picked up my first book on the workings of the brain, and within a short time, the subject had me hooked. (Right now I'm working myself through two books: *Living with Our Genes: Why They Matter More Than You Think*, written by Dean Hamer and Peter Copeland, published in 1998 by Doubleday, and *A User's Guide to the Brain: Perception, Attention and the Four Theaters of the Brain*, written by John J. Ratey, published in 2001 by Pantheon Books.)

I have already shared in the Definitions section a little of what I have learned about the brain and will return to the subject shortly. But I will begin with a few words about genes and the immune system. Maybe it will entice you to look at these fascinating subjects in more depth. After all, it's not said for naught that MS persons are a strong, intelligent and knowledge-thirsty bunch.

When you read about MS, especially in the area of research, you will come across words and phrases like "genetically caused disease," "autoimmune disease," "viral theory," "the immune system." For some time, I was satisfied with having a basic understanding of what people and the print media were talking about, but the finer points eluded me. It seemed they were too round for my square head. Well, one day—oh blessed event—I was alone in the house for a couple of hours. I got my two MS Bibles out—the Rosner-Ross and the Lechtenberg books—

plus assorted dictionaries and encyclopedias and decided I'd figure that bleepetybleep immune system out once and for all. So for all of you who are a little fuzzy and puzzled, here's what I came up with, and I present you with this unscientific, layperson view of how things work.

Oh, for the basics on genetics, I have to thank our CR for a fantastic introductory article, and my grandniece, who borrowed a biology book from her high school and let me wade through it till I got it—at least sort of, I hope. No, I'm not there yet, not by a long shot, but I keep on reading and making margin notes.

The Genes and MS

I was awed by the number of neurons, their connections and interconnections in the brain. Well, looking at the field of genetics is even more mind boggling.

Try to picture this:

There are trillions of cells in the body, and in each cell are twenty-three pairs of chromosomes. Inside the chromosomes are the hundreds of thousands of genes. The genes contain the whole individuality blueprint of a person and nudge the cells to produce certain proteins.

Well, as I make mistakes transposing my handwritten notes onto the computer screen, so does the body make occasional typographical errors. I can edit my output and correct the mistakes, but the body doesn't have a spell checker; it sends out faulty genes which can contribute to the eruption of certain diseases. If the carrier of that defective gene becomes a parent, he or she sends half of her or his genes on to her or his child, and the runts could be among the bunch.

Now here is the doozie: Most genetically-caused diseases are caused by a single gene, but we MSers have to be different and make the game of hide and seek more hide than find on those trying to find out about us. As Dr. Rammohan said, there are at least four genes responsible (one research note I found in 2002 said more like twenty are now under consideration) for MS development, and it is harder to find our pattern, this combination of several genes. (I just wonder, are they bunched together and presented to the child en bloc ?)

75

But if the genes thought they could hide out forever and not be discovered so they could continue to make some people feel miserable, ha, they have another think coming. Scientists aren't discouraged, and major grants from the National to fund projects most certainly will help in ferreting the rascal out.

The Immune System and MS

The immune system is that part of (or in) us which is supposed to ward off, fight off and kill off foreign invaders that enter our bodies, something that can make us ill if these trespassers are allowed to do their dirty work. Stress, poor health, depression are some of the things which can weaken the immune system so it can't do its job properly.

Let me just recall and expand on a few items from the glossary, words you will frequently hear or read when the immune system is being discussed:

T-Lymphocytes or simply T-cells: They are one type of white blood cells, have a hand in and play a role in producing antibodies, which in our case eat away the myelin which leads to lesion formation which distorts messages or completely hinders nerve impulses from reaching their destination, which causes MS symptoms.

These T-cells come in different varieties—Killer, Helper and Suppressor. Of great interest are the Suppressor T-cells. They are supposed to tell the Killer cells to stop, but as I said in the Definitions, as our kids sometimes don't listen to us, some cells don't listen to the immune system either.

Antigen: That's the aggressor that likes to make a person sick and does make us sick when the immune system isn't working right. Normally the appearance of an antigen leads to the birth of the accurate antibody, the T and B cells but...

Antibody: It is supposed to attack foreign invaders, but in MS, it attacks the myelin instead, ratfink that it is. You might have been told that the lab found gamma globulin in your spinal fluid. That belongs to the family of antibodies and shows that your body is fighting off an inflammation or infection or a virus.

Isn't it utterly amazing though how orderly our different body systems are working with each other? How one is intertwined with another? How one depends on the other?

Even in cases where this working hand-in-glove is detrimental to said body owner's health, everything is well-orchestrated.

Autoimmune Diseases

Besides multiple sclerosis, lupus, rheumatoid arthritis, some ulcers and Graves disease are also autoimmune diseases.

In the normal-working immune system, the lymphocytes (B and T-cells) go in cohorts with macrophages (scavenger cells) and produce antibodies to defeat antigens. The antibodies jump on the bad cells and try to kill 'em dead in order to keep the body in halfway decent working order.

In autoimmune diseases, though, the antibodies don't attack the intruders but attack the body's own healthy cells.

Researchers concentrate their attention on the immune system to find out what makes it tick and try to find out how they can set the wayward child on the path of righteousness. A lot has already been discovered, but lots more work needs to be done. In the end, the separate pieces need to be gathered together and compiled to a whole.

Viral Theory of Causes for MS

Some MS researchers speculate that a virus may have sneaked in during a person's teenage years, or an old one may have stayed behind, having somehow survived, hiding out till awakened by the Factor X trigger.

(I have spent at least five hours on the computer, trying to find updated research data, but I was not very successful in discovering more than I had found out up to 1996. But neither has anything I had written then been disproved.)

As far as I know, no specific virus has been blamed, but it is being said that it may be a quite common rascal—like the one that causes cold sores, the herpes virus (HHV-6) or the one that causes German measles (rubella).

For a time, the measles virus was singled out for special attention and was, rather still is, thought to be in some way responsible for the onset of MS. In most people, the measles virus causes only measles, and the body produces antibodies to snare it if it should come around again. But it is conjectured that in an elite group—us MSers—one or a few of them may have survived the T-lymphocyte onslaught.

I have read about a new theory. Maybe, it is being said, a person who has the susceptibility to develop MS (genetically speaking) may not handle a viral infection as well as a person who doesn't have the flawed genes and the Factor X trigger (or, as I have heard it being called, an environmental influence) can start having its heyday.

It is a fact, though, that researchers explore if that certain, as of now, unknown virus is granted safe harbor by the oligodentrocytes, the very cells which produce the myelin that is being destroyed, eaten away and replaced with MS plaques.

I have read another interesting piece a while ago. It suggested that maybe the virus hides in the myelin and the immune system attacks it to kill the virus. Now wouldn't that make the most sense? I just wonder why it has not been followed up. (At least I have not heard anything about it.)

Besides common viruses that are considered in the search for cause and cure of multiple sclerosis, researchers have found one specific virus in MS persons, called human T-cell lymphotropic virus-1, HTLV-1 for short. The discovery of that virus caused some fear and confusion in MS persons and the general population alike, because of the similarity of HTLV-1 and HIV—human immunodeficiency virus, associated with AIDS. I want to stress strongly and emphatically, and you ought to do so too, should anybody hint at MS being in the same category as AIDS. MS is nothing at all like AIDS. The two are completely different diseases.

However it is handled, the viral theory states that a virus may be in the body, hides out, tickles the immune system into doing some minor damage (or as I heard and read recently, it causes leaks in the Blood Brain Barrier, which lets the virus or the Myelin Basic Protein into the brain proper) and then prepares for the Big Attack.

In November 2003, I read reports and saw postings on bulletin boards that said that a new avenue was being explored, it having to do with iron deposits in the brain and that not only the white matter of the brain (the myelinated nerve fibers), but also the gray matter (the unmyelinated nerve fibers) are involved in the vandalism. I do hope you have access to a computer and can check out for yourself how much is being done.

One diagnosis note: It is a well-known fact that many people with clear MS-signs remain in the undiagnosed, the probable, the potential category, because the clinical evidence is not provable. (In the meantime, they are unable to avail themselves to the injectables that everybody suggests the MSer should get on to as soon as the diagnosis is established. Grrrrr on over-cautious doctors!)

At the same time I learned about the iron deposits, I also read about a new or additional method of diagnosis, it being a blood test, to see if the lab can find garbage in the blood, you know, the litter from the inflammation or the nerve cells or the immune system stuff. This, it is being said, may speed up the diagnosis.

About time, I'd say, don't you think?

My Summary

Okay, here is how I think MS is getting started and how it is kept going:

A. A couple of genes are faulty.

B. A virus stays active, or a new one sneaks in during a specifically dangerous time in a person's life—teenage years are mentioned most frequently.

C. Whatever it is, it hides out somewhere.

D. The Factor X trigger awakens the virus or nudges the genes to attack a minor or unimportant area to let the person know it is there.

E. Eventually the bugger (the Factor X trigger, I mean) gets impatient; it pulls the wool over the immune system's eyes, ears and nose, cries "wolf" to the white blood cells and sends them on the rampage to happily gnaw away our good myelin. Result: Lesions, plagues, MS symptoms.

I'll end this segment with a joke I've heard and even can remember, probably because we hear so often how good we look or sound.

A woman comes to the doctor and talks about her symptoms that bother her a lot. "But you look so good," says the good doctor.

The woman repeats her tale of woe and is once again told that she looks so good. She gets impatient. "Why shouldn't I?" she snaps. "I'm not sick in the face."

Research

HTLV-1: I have mentioned this virus a moment ago but would like to expand on it a bit.

In the late 1980s/early 1990s, another flurry of excitement swept through TV, newspapers, and our support group members. The virus which causes MS has been discovered! Hurrah, hurrah and hurray!! Every MS person will be healed within the next forty-eight hours!!!

At least so the media implied.

Of course that was nothing but another case of exaggerated hype. The National responded with the statement that a Swedish group of scientists had extended the research that they had already reported on three years earlier. Using more sophisticated equipment, they found a "relationship between a retrovirus (HTLV-1) and MS. It does not imply that the retrovirus is the cause of MS." Further on, the National's memo stated: "The recent data have infused a new excitement into research on multiple sclerosis."

"It cannot be stressed enough that there is no connection between MS and AIDS.

"A press release from the Wistar Institute comments: 'Although HTLV-1 and the AIDS virus HIV are related, they are distinctly different viruses. People infected with HTLV-1, including those with MS, are in absolutely no danger of developing AIDS.'"

I would amend that statement with "…are in no danger of developing AIDS unless they acquire the HIV virus."

I want to add here that during a study conducted by the Ohio Department of Health, it was found that HTLV-1 levels were slightly higher in "cases than controls." I will report on this study in detail later on but thought you might keep it in the back of your mind.

MSWGMD

In the 1996 edition of this book, I wrote the following:

Over the last couple of months, I have read about cladribine therapy and the magazine *Real Living with MS* (Volume 2, Number 7, June 1995, published by the Cobb Group) had an extensive article on the pros and cons of this therapy. Dr. Labe Scheinberg suggested to an MS patient, she try experimentally the drug which is FDA-approved as a chemotherapy for hairy cell leukemia. [I have no idea what that could be, do you?] Most people in the small group who had been given cladribine did well, and Dr. Scheinberg's patient, too, had her symptoms of chronic-progressive MS arrested.

On the other hand, the article noted the objections of Dr. Ernest Beutler; he urged a "wait for test results first" approach.

Ortho Biotech though had trials at several cities going on and requested volunteers contact their 800 number to request information.

On 23 March 2002, I went to the Google Search Engine, asked for "cladribine therapy for multiple sclerosis" and received an astonishing amount of links. On the website *canjneurolsci.org*, I found out that clinical trials must have continued in the intervening years, that cladribine, taken by chronic progressive MS patients, was well tolerated. I also found out that cladribine has immunosuppressive effects, that the results are encouraging but more information is needed before conclusions can be drawn. (Oh bleepetybleep grrrr, how I hate that delaying mechanism.)

I do learn from visits at bulletin boards that it seems chemotherapy is used more frequently now with good results.

But in 1996, something else peeked my interest regarding this subject. I called our local library for the correct spelling of "Human T-cell Lymphotropic Virus" (HLTV-1) and any info they could find for me. The librarian told me that HTLV-3 is associated with leukemia. I don't know if that is only for hairy cell leukemia or leukemia per se. As I said, cladribine is approved for leukemia treatment and is also tried on people with multiple sclerosis.

Can we say "Aha" already or be satisfied with a "Hm?"

MSWGMD

In the February 1990 issue of the *Reader's Digest* magazine I read an interesting item in their "News From Medicine" column, titled "New drug boost transplant odds." It talked about the anti-rejection drug FK506. Since MS is mentioned in connection with this drug, I asked the National for more information, and they sent me Memo # 355-89, dated February 7, 1989.

As I understand it, FK506 constitutes an improvement over cyclosporine and is hundreds of times more powerful than cyclosporine. You may have heard cyclosporine has already been investigated for use in certain types of MS, but because it has too many serious side effects, the tests were halted.

(The material I found in the beginning of March 2002 stated that cyclosporine was still being investigated.)

Here is the basic information from Memo 355-89:

FK506 is a new immunosuppressive drug (that is, in our case, it is supposed to make the immune system stop mistaking its host body's myelin as a foreign invader), used experimentally in organ transplant surgery. It is supposed to replace cyclosporine, and the author of the memo talked about "superior performance" and said that "initial studies look promising." But he pointed out that FK506 definitely has fewer side effects and offers the potential of a more effective and safer treatment for certain types of MS.

In the early or mid-90s, I read in a newspaper that FK506 was used in one major transplant case and that the patient was doing quite well.

So far I could not find anything newer on this subject. I think it might have been renamed in the meantime.

MSWGMD

In *Inside MS*, Vol. 8, # 4, Fall 1990, I read the first article on efforts to remyelinate the MS scars. The title: "Transplanting Oligo; Object: To replace the myelin sheath."

This means that by now, research in this area has been going on for twelve years, right? Wouldn't one think they would have come up with something concrete or at least something a little more substantial?

I found another research item in another *Inside MS* issue (Vol. 9, #1, Winter 1991). Teresa Doolittle and her colleagues at Massachusetts General Hospital undertook a study to find out if autoimmune diseases run in families. Their conclusion? "Yes, of course they do, because susceptibility can be inherited."

You notice, this was stated as a factual conclusion. So why in bleepetybleep do they still deny it? I won't belabor the point again about proud offsprings receiving chromosomes from proud parents, but I mean, duh...come on...

MSWGMD

It may appear that the information gleaned from Memo #264, dated October 12, 1990, about a neurologists' meeting may be thought of as having been superceded by newer information—I'm sure there have been other neurologists' meeting since 1990
that resulted in a presentation of exciting discoveries—but I found this one item particularly interesting. The presentation provided results of studies regarding the use of Magnetic Resonance Imaging (MRI)

Investigators from the Institute of Neurological Disorders and Stroke (their website is fantastic) observed MS patients who were believed to be in remission. These patients underwent monthly MRI scans. Along with clinical exams, the present scans were being compared with the ones from the previous month.

Now hear this: Even though the people did not show any new symptoms, nor a worsening of their condition or other disease activities, the MRI showed new lesions! (Proves again to me what an absolutely impressive number of nerve cells are in the brain; not all of them are used, but I venture a guess that some could be pulled into action if some others were demyelinated.)

But you know what angers me? If I hadn't been an officer in the support group, hadn't asked for that particular research material and read it carefully, I would never have found out about all this. In other words, doesn't it seem as if somebody wants to keep us uninformed? Or do they think we're not smart enough to understand complex issues? Or do they fear somebody would steal their thunder? Or maybe another scientist could build on their material and get results faster?

Grrr, dang it, that really irks me—and yeah, yeah, yeah, I'll get off my soap box and tell you about another MRI item.

A Canadian group proved that point through another MRI study. Lesions in both exacerbation-remission as well as chronic-progressive types of MS were studied, and they found no difference in MS activities in the two groups. The clinicians concluded that all MS is progressive, even while the person is in the undiagnosed state or is in clinical remission.

MSWGMD

Will you join me in some thinking and reasoning? Maybe you will come up with different ideas, rebuke me or agree with me? Well, here is how I see it.

The MSers in the exacerbation-remission group have flare-ups of varying length and severity. That's the time when old symptoms get worse or new ones appear. After it is over, a blessed remission grants a sense of feeling relatively well or at least a bit better.

The findings in Memo #264, though, say that the Factor X trigger doesn't snooze but wants to be continually fed by the immune system. (Does he/she/it feel like the queen bee whose worker bees have to supply her with, I believe it's nectar?) Thus the immune system continues to perform its sneaky crime of constantly purloining our myelin.

Okay, those are the basics. Now the analyzing. This is how I envision it: Faulty genes have weakened the response of the immune system to a certain virus which has stayed behind or creeps in during a particularly vulnerable time in the person's life. (The teenage years are mentioned prominently.) The bad kid on the block, the Factor X trigger (environmental, trauma, stress, poor general health, heat and humidity), wakes up or gets mad; it goes on the prowl, bullies or misleads the immune system into seeing the myelin as an antigen which needs to be eliminated. Antibodies are produced which are supposed to destroy the perceived enemy. These antibodies swim along in the bloodstream which nourishes the brain and gnaw holes in our myelin.

Or consider another scenario: Maybe the antibodies poke holes into the Blood Brain Barrier to provide an opening for the antibodies, the Myelin Basic Protein, to enter and do their dirty work.

My question is this: Is the Factor X trigger the slavedriver who doesn't let the immune system rest? Or is he/she/it misleading the immune system as to where an attack is needed? Or couldn't it be that the suppressor T-cells are duped from knowing when enough is enough and makes them believe the danger is permanent and thus they have to continue to produce and reproduce like insects?

MSWGMD

In 1995, our CR sent me an undated clipping. Ann Futterman of the University of Colorado Health Center conducted a study, funded by the Norman Cousin Foundation, on the effect of strong emotions. She of course discovered—*tatah*—that they do influence the number of "natural killer cells" which stand health-guard and greet unwanted invaders by killing them.

Please don't say that's not a nice way to greet a guest. You wouldn't invite a robber into you house or welcome somebody with a baseball bat who you know wants to hit your legs away from under you, nor be hospitable to somebody who you know would do you harm, now would you?

Anyway, these study-findings give permission to get angry, pound the table or jump for joy—even if you, like me, can only do it mentally—and see what it does for you. There is only one thing you are not allowed to do, and that is giving up. And don't you think these strong emotions activate and increase the endorphins?

Dr. Cedric Raine and Eae

I wrote this in 1996:

> Neuroimmunologist Dr. Raine has been on the forefront of MS research for thirty years. In fact, according to *Inside MS* (vol. 14, no. 2, Summer 1996) "he has devoted his career to MS research and has written more than 330 publications on MS" and made excellent strides in discovering what is going on in MS persons' bodies. Deservedly so, he won the 1996 John Dystel Award. (Mr. Dystel was a lawyer who had MS, and his family created this award in his honor in 1994.)
>
> In this *Inside MS* issue is a condensed report of Dr. Raine's work—from oligos to macrophages to myelin to remyelination. (I hope the National has made this report a Fact Sheet.) This article details Dr. Raine's accomplishments and puts scientific terms into language understandable by laypersons.
>
> Here I want to speak mainly about Experimental Allergic Encephalomyelitis, EAE for short. [I have read some call it "Experimental Autoimmune Encephalomyelitis"; I don't know when and why the original name has been changed. I will continue to use the designation I see used most recently.]
>
> EAE is a demyelinating disease induced in animals. It acts very much like multiple sclerosis in humans and helps researchers to eventually help us. Following are some EAE highlights.

Inside MS carried an article about remyelination (vol. 9, # 1, Winter 1990). Its title: "Rebuilding Myelin from Scratch" and constitutes an interview with Dr. Raine. He said in this particular interview that investigators have seen extensive remyelination and now work with animals to test theories on how to induce remyelination in human multiple sclerosis patients. In 1990, they had already achieved some promising results. Eventually they will feel confident enough to progress to human beings.

Dr. Raine has conducted research on MS-damaged brains (of course these people were dead) and also on the EAE-afflicted animals. I don't know how he concocted the Myelin Basic Protein brew, nor do I know how he was able to help them toward a remyelination, remission or recovery of the animals; all I know is that he did develop the right mixture of the right ingredients to inject in the animals with the desired results, and they had no further flare-ups. In fact, a few of the symptoms disappeared.

As I said, this appeared in the 1996 edition. Here is the update for 2002:

Dr. Raine's webpage says he is a neuropathologist. He was and is with the Einstein College of Medicine. It lists an abundance of research projects he is or was engaged in. (I wonder if he has discovered the forty-eight-hour day with only a few hours of sleep necessary to get all that accomplished.) I would say if anybody finds something concrete, it will be Dr. Raine. Although, he too will have to deal with the exorbitant (that means excessive time- and money-consuming) regulations of the Food and Drug Administration (FDA) and pharmaceutical houses interested in their bottom line and investor's dividends.

MSWGMD

Research Report 102/91 (dated May 17, 1991) talks about mitoxantrone, an immunosuppressive drug which has helped mice sick with EAE. It was tested for safety in a small trial on chronic-progressive MS patients. Well, the MSers didn't get any worse and had only a few side effects which doctors could easily alleviate.

But here is the clincher: Dr. Noseworthy of the Mayo Clinic in Rochester, MN, said mitoxantrone "may be a candidate for a full trial."

Update: Mitoxantrone is listen as "experimental therapy." I don't know how far trials have advanced or if the medication is already dispensed on an experimental basis.

MSWGMD

A few new or refresher glossary items:

Antigen and Antibody: The antigen, that foreign invader, thief, robber, whatever you want to call that what makes people ill, enters the body. It carries its personal marker, the lock. An antibody, specifically geared toward sniffing out this one particular antigen, is the key; it locks onto the antigen and tries its best to, alone or with assistance to eliminate the intruder.
Astrocytes: They manufacture the stuff that forms the scar tissue which covers the lesions which bring on MS symptoms…well, you know all about that already, more than you care for, right?
Cytokines: They are responsible for growth or death of cells.
Myelin Basic Protein (MBP): That is the debris, the fragments of myelin, white blood cells and so on, which either penetrate the blood-brain barrier or leak into the spinal fluid
Oligodentrocytes, the Oligos: They manufacture the myelin.
Tumor Necrosis Factor, the TNF: It is able to deprive a tumor of its blood supply and kills it dead.

Scar Trek is the title of a report in another issue of *Inside MS* (Vol. 9, # 4, Fall/Winter 1991). Dr. Etty Benveniste investigated "the interaction between cells of the immune system and cells of the brain" and works with EAE-resistant and EAE-susceptible animals. She studied cytokines and asked what, if any, effect cytokines had on oligos and astrocytes.

She specifically studied one type of cytokines, the tumor necrosis factor, and found TNF not only kills tumors, but also different types of cells.

The Summer 1996 issue of *Inside MS* (the one that talked about Dr. Cedric Raine) mentions that Dr. Raine also works, among other things, on oligos and TNF.

MSWGMD

The *Mayo Clinic Health Letter* talks about on-going research, for instance Intravenous Immunoglobulin (IVIg) which takes antibodies from healthy donors and injects them into people who have MS, trying to stimulate myelin-producing cells. They also try plasma exchanges. They take "factors which are believed to be involved in immune attacks" and replace them with new plasma.

Update of 2002: Both of the above two items are listed, among many others, as "experimental therapy."

MSWGMD

On July 30, 1996, our local newspaper, the *Galion Inquirer*, carried a small Associated Press item, titled Gene Hunters Close in on Inherited MS Factors. It said that scientists have come one step closer to finding the genes which predispose some people to develop multiple sclerosis and cited Margaret Perical-Vance, a genetic researcher at Duke University Medical Center in Durham, NC.

But I snorted, snickered and harrumphed at the short final paragraph that cautioned that these studies did not show that MS is an inherited disease.

No comment of mine required, right? I don't want my blood pressure to top out again.

MSWGMD

In the beginning of November 2003, I read and heard several reports about MS persons receiving marijuana (cannabis) in pill form. I don't know if that was a smaller or larger test group and whether that was experimental or what. Neither have I heard anything about side effects. All I have heard is that the participants reported relief from their MS symptoms.

Treatments and Medications

I will start with the story of the interferons; that is, the story of Betaseron, Avonex, Copaxone and Rebif. Betaseron: I didn't pay much attention to the interferons until 1992. Sure, I had heard rumors about something being in the works, something MS-specific, something that was supposed to reduce the numbers of exacerbations an MS person had to endure. That sounded exciting, but I was leery about it, remembering what Dr. Rammohan from the OSU Clinics had said about interferon's toxicity.

By March 2002, I had learned that interferons are natural proteins, produced by the body to fight off infections—which brings my one-track-mind back to all the questions about the Factor X trigger, wondering what kind of a virus the betas are fighting and what its role is, whether it is a common, well known one, one that causes other illnesses (like measles or cold sores) and just acts different in people who develop multiple sclerosis or if it is an MS-specific one which has so far escaped detection? Or is it the virus who pokes holes in the Blood-Brain Barrier for the gunkjunk to get inside the brain proper? Dang it, it's all so bleepetybleep frustrating!

Anyway, back to the interferons. In the June 1992 support group meeting, our treasurer told us that she had been contacted by a lady who was part of a nationwide lobbying group, trying to urge the FDA to give preferential treatment to the approval of beta interferon.

The lady had included a packet of explanatory letters and petitions, to be signed and forwarded to Dr. Kessler, the then-FDA administrator. Our treasurer had already taken the packet to her campground and had gathered thirty-eight signatures. The sixteen attendees of the meeting signed their copies, and when my daughter came to pick me up, we asked her to sign too, but she begged off, saying she wanted to think about it and talk with me first.

And talk she did, giving up her precious sleep (she worked two jobs and had a family to take care of) and motivated me to widen the petition drive to a personal letter-writing campaign, "making it a message of human interest," she said. The letters could be mailed to the President, area and national law makers, major newspapers, TV stations and the like.

Well, I sacrificed some of my sleep, too, drafted the letter and typed it the next morning. With the help of one at the ladies of the public library, I had copies made, got the addresses and sent out forty-eight letters with the FDA Petition attached. (Our local newspaper, the *Galion Inquirer*, granted me permission to reprint some of my "Letters to the Editor" in this book. You can find a few samples in the appendix. Maybe they will give you ideas for a letter-writing campaign of your own.)

Let me tell you, it worked. The FDA admitted they were overwhelmed. They had never experienced such an outpouring of a response. The FDA Advisory Committee recommended approval; in July 1993, the FDA gave its consent; beta interferon 1b was named Betaseron, and soon afterwards, it hit the pharmacy shelves. After an initial shortage, the supply stabilized and became widely available to anyone who wanted it. Rather I should say it became available to anybody who could afford it.

Well, all I can say is that *we did it* and can move on to the next project. At least the FDA knows we are out here and can make our voices heard.

Avonex: And guess what, Avonex, another MS-specific drug, ran the concourse much quicker. On May 18, 1996, our *Galion Inquirer* printed a lengthy Associated Press story of Avonex, the second self-administered injectable MS-drug, having been approved.

It did not go as smoothly though. Berlex Industries, who manufacture Betaseron announced they would seek an injunction to ban Biogen, the manufacturer of Avonex from distributing the drug, citing the Orphan Drug Act. (It grants companies a financial reward and marketing exclusivity for developing drugs for rare diseases.) Berlex claimed Avonex (beta 1a) was too close in composition and applicability to Betaseron (beta 1b).

A few days later (July 30, 1996) I heard on the CNN Headline News financial segment that Biogen's stock had risen due to the sale of an MS drug. This led me to believe that Avonex was now on the market. It was.

Now the story of number three:

Cop-1: In the late 1980s, copolymer-1 was much in the news and, as I said earlier, was already prescribed in Israel. Our chairperson wrote to the Baylor College of Medicine in Houston, TX, which was in charge of the research of this specific area. Here is a copy of the answer she received:

> The study of copolymer-1 in patients with chronic-progressive MS has been concluded but unfortunately the results were not very satisfactory. While there were some people in the study who improved and did quite well on the treatment, others apparently were not benefitted and the overall results were not sufficiently beneficial to recommend its use at this time…
>
> …further studies are being designed and we hope to continue studying it and getting more information about it. It will probably not be available in the near future…

Like many of our group members, I was disappointed that another hope had been dashed, but as I said in the newsletter, we all can hope that something else will be discovered—and soon.

Then, *tatah*, *Inside MS* (vol. 9, Spring 1991) reported that clinical trials on cop-1 had been started up again. It had been discovered that cop-1 suppresses EAE in animals and was thought to be beneficial for the exacerbation-remission type of MS.

A short note, in Spring 1993, spoke of cop-1's clinical trials going on at several locations across the country.

In the Winter/Spring issue of *Inside MS*, I read that TEVA Pharmaceutical Industries in Israel and Kulpsville, PA, work on cop-1. It will be named Copaxon, will be another medication administered via injections under the skin (subcutaneously, as they call it) and is supposed to decrease the numbers of exacerbations an MS person experiences.

Oh, a neat item appeared in the Chapter's Winter 1995 *MS Relay*, the Northwest Ohio Chapter's official magazine. It said Teva Pharmaceuticals USA was looking for volunteers to participate in a cop-1 study. I call it guinea pigging and would gladly do it, but, well, read on.

Guess what the prerequisites for this so-called volunteering was: The participant had to shell out $7,300; that is, seven thousand, three hundred dollars a year for the medication, in addition to taking on the risk entailed in the endeavor, since they were double-blind studies, not knowing whether one received the real thing or the placebo. But no matter which one the guinea pig received, the cost was still $7,300 a year.

Well, kind and gentle reader, I blew my top in, *uh*, very strong emotions and language. Normally I cuss in German, people don't understand what I'm saying and think I'm such a good girl who doesn't use bad language, but once or twice a year, I do the cussing in American words. Every two or three years even the "f" word floats past my otherwise sweet lips. In ninety percent of the cases, it's the FDA that provokes such outbreaks, not only because of the slowness in medication approval, but also because of their stand on tobacco products. I'm a smoker, don't feel guilty about it, don't try to quit; all my doctors know it and have given up chastising me about it.

Okay, stop sidetracking yourself Elvira K. and watch your blood pressure.

Anyway, after reading that snippet, I fired off another letter to the *Galion Inquirer*. You can find the copy of that one in the Appendix too.

Well, after all that haggling, on September 20, 1996, I heard on the CNN News (Current News Network out of Atlanta, GA) that the FDA Advisory Committee recommended that copolymer-1 (Copaxon) be approved for multiple sclerosis patients who suffered from a mild to moderate course of the disease.

Since most of the Advisory Committee's recommendations are accepted, Copaxon was approved.

Now there were three, but sometime in 2002, Rebif was approved for distribution. I don't know much about it, but since it is an interferon 1a, it shouldn't be too different from Avonex. I believe it is or was manufactured in Great Britain. I also seem to recall that I heard Rebif's composition is somewhat stronger, and it is injected three times a week instead of once a week for Avonex.

MSWGMD

In 1996, I wrote in the newsletter: Personally I'm still waiting for something cheaper and especially waiting for something I can take by mouth. I could never give myself shots.

As I said, that was in 1996. Do you remember that snippet about me and the computers and the chiropractor (to be discussed shortly) or any of the other areas where I said "I'll never..." Well, I'll tell you in a moment how this specific never changed in September 2000.

MSWGMD

I will end this segment with the wish that I could tell you of all the exciting news I have found on the Internet about research findings and new medications being in the pipelines, in trials and already prescribed as experimental treatments. Since the information found on the Internet is copyright-protected though, I do hope you will find a way to find out about it. I am sure it will raise your hopes too. Just click on to your favorite search engine, type the words "Multiple sclerosis research" or "Multiple sclerosis medications" and see what a wealth of news and interesting links you will come up with.

Now I will shut the monitor off for a while, get me a coffee cup refill, smoke me a cigarette and relax.

Well, I did the three things, took my shot, and since it was elevenish, I decided to fix an early lunch (two scrambled eggs and an English muffin with jelly) since I only had a half of a banana flip for breakfast.

Yes, I'm baching it at the moment and eat whatever I want when I want it—and those aren't nutritious meals with all the four food groups.

And since April 2003 (since my husband's death), my cupboards have been filled with sweets and snacks and the freezer with TV dinners.

Medications (oral)

Here is what I am personally familiar with.

Lioresal—generic name baclofen—is an anti-spasticity medication. According to my pharmacy's leaflet, it is prescribed primarily for multiple sclerosis and spinal cord injuries. For me it works, limbers up the limbs and makes movements easier.

Normally I take the prescribed amount—20 mg three to four times a day—but when I know I have to be on my feet for a while, I skip one dose or take a half one. Sometimes I want to be a little stiffish. I've been taking Lioresal since I was diagnosed with MS in 1982. (Yes, I had my twenty-year anniversary and still walk and talk and think and read and write.)

Symmetrel—generic name amantadine—is an anti-viral medication, supposed to aid in nerve conduction. It is also supposed to aid in the alleviation of fatigue. An added benefit is the fact that I haven't had a serious cold or the flu since I started taking it. Zanaflex, another of the newer drugs on the market, falls in the same category. I've taken amantadine practically since I'm diagnosed, but my neurologist takes me off for three to six weeks now and then to prevent my body from getting too used to it and having it stop being effective.

For a while I took the anti-depressant Elavil—generic name amytriptyline. In addition to lifting depression, it is also supposed to act as a pain medication for MS patients. After a couple of years, I told the neurologist I wanted to stop it because I had read some bad publicity. I also had a fear of addiction, especially after I met an MS person who was hooked on Valium and desperately went from doctor to doctor, trying to get more prescriptions. That is the reason why I would never accede to taking Valium or Lithium—and that is a never I will never break.

But a couple of years ago, I gave in to my doctor and let him prescribe an anti-depressant for me. The first three did not work. One made me snappy, mean-spirited and aggressive, which is not me; the other didn't do anything, and the third, well, I just didn't like the side effects. So we experimented with Celexa, and that does just fine for me. (That's why I appreciate my neurologist so much; he realizes I know what is right for me and lets me set the tone of my medical care.)

Every two to three years, I also take the oral cortico steroid regime— Prednisone—and it does a lot of good.

(By now my osteo- and rheumatoid arthritis require me to take an NSAID, a non-steroidal anti-inflammatory drug.)

I do know of MSers who take Tegretol for face pain. Our treasurer and a friend were being helped with Dilantin for energy and tremors.

I hear and read a lot about Neurontin (taken orally, a strong pain reliever) and Solu-Medrol (a steroid treatment, given intravenously at home) and Provigil. I looked up the medications on the Internet, but since I have no experience and don't know anybody who takes them, I would rather not comment; what I read on the bulletin boards is somewhat contradictory—some people think it helps them, while others talk about side effect and so on. If you are interested, please check with your pharmacist or medical personnel.

MSWGMD

Okay, now a bit more about the new kids on the block. I found this information on the Merck-Medco website. The purpose for all four injectables is to decrease the frequency of exacerbations and delay onset of disability.

Betaseron: Interferon Beta 1b. It is an anti-viral, injected under the skin every other day. Please check with other Betaseron-users or on an MS bulletin board regarding side effects.

Copaxone: The copolymer-1 derivative. It is designed specifically for use in MS patients. It is injected daily under the skin. If you should consider getting a prescription for Copaxone, please check with other Copaxone-users for side effects.

Avonex: This interferon Beta 1a is an anti-viral and immune-regulatory drug. It is injected into the muscle once a week.

Rebif: Another interferon Beta 1a, ergo an anti-viral and immune regulatory drug. It is injected three times a week under the skin.

Okay, I can talk about Avonex from experience and do so to anybody. I like it. It is good. It helps me. Here is another one of my "I'll never..." stories.

I had always bragged that my neurologist (yes, the one I want to clone because I think he's the best) didn't even mention the ABCs. Well, in September 2000, he aggravated me, asked me to consider going on Avonex. I hemmed and hawed about being afraid to give myself a shot and that I didn't believe I needed it and that I was afraid. Did he urge me to change my mind? Nope, he just (dang him) said: "Would you rather be in a wheelchair in the future, being unable to do things or join your family in outings?"

Well, I begged for time to acquaint myself with the thought; he gave me my prescription for the other four medications I take and told me to give his office a call if or when I changed my mind.

Well, I mulled it over and over and over. Finally I called the office and told the nurse, "Okay, I'll try it." A few days later, the prescription arrived in the mail. I called my insurance company, hoping they'd say, no, they didn't cover it because it was so expensive, but the cheerful lady said, "Oh yes, it is covered in your plan." Dang it. Well, I sent that little piece of paper off with the required co-payment, and a few days later, the ice chest arrived with three packages in it. I put the three boxes in my icebox and mulled some more. And then thought again. And considered it another time for good (or was it bad) measure.

By that time it was November, and I decided to call the Avonex Helpline. The kindest young lady spoke with me, and her encouraging words gave me the power to call my daughter-in-law and ask her if she were willing to train me. Of course she said yes, and Sunday afternoon she and my son appeared at my door. He disappeared in the living room to join his father, leaving us girls in the kitchen. My daughter-in-law gave me some background, opened that package and neatly laid out the contents—syringe, needle, two alcohol wipes, sterile gauze pad, band aid and two small bottles, one with liquid, one with a white powder. Efficiently she mixed the liquid with the powder, explaining each step, and then gave me the shot. "Hey, there's really nothing to it," I had to exclaim, and she agreed.

Well, the next Sunday she once again performed the ritual, and for two Sundays after that, she had me do it. I almost did it right the first time, only forgot to wipe the bottle tops with the alcohol pad before inserting the needle.

On the fifth Sunday, she was detained, and, heart pounding, I went through the steps myself and successfully gave myself my first unsupervised injection. Was I proud? Yes. As I had said, there was nothing to it. Did side effects bother me? I had been warned that I may feel flu-like symptoms, but I followed my neurologist's advise, took two Tylenol on the shot morning and two before bed time and was just fine.

But here is the funny thing. I still have Sunday set up as my shot day. On Friday night or Saturday morning, I start sniffling and sneezing, have headaches and a runny nose. As soon as I take the shot, I'm fine again. In other words, I have the side effects which I am supposed to have after the shot before the shot. Oh well, I have been told several times that I'm weird. (For instance, I like my yogurt with whipped cream under and lots of sugar on top, and one of my sisters-in-law finds that weird.)

Now since the beginning of October 2003, Avonex comes in pre-filled syringes. All I need to do is assemble needle and vial, wipe my leg with the alcohol pad, give the shot, hold the gauze pad and affix the band aid—all provided—and am good for another week.

Also, a few days ago, I read about a study/report that warned about neutralizing antibodies that decrease the effectiveness of the beta interferons. But guess what, Avonex had the lowest incidence.

MSWGMD

The husband of one of our group members was the son of a chiropractor and talked frequently about the benefits of chiropractic.

Well, I shook my head and inwardly told myself that I'd never go to see one of them.... Yes, in my thoughts I used the nasty description often heard. How soon would I have to eat my words.

Another one of our group members often swore that after months of being bed ridden, it was acupuncture that got him into a remission and back on his feet. (This gentleman was in his seventies, was diagnosed with MS for quite some time, but walked only with a cane and really got around very well.)

Well, on January 2, 1991, I caught a program on the Discovery Channel. The reporter talked about acupuncture and said, among other benefits, acupuncture also induced and stimulated the production of endorphins.

Uh, well, endorphins, hm? I passed that on to the group, and our treasurer insisted that endorphin production was stimulated much more by laughter, which, she insisted, was another MS treatment. To help with inducing laughter, she proceeded to tell a couple of jokes.

1. Old folks are worth a fortune. They have silver in their hair, gold in their teeth, stones in their kidneys, lead in their feet and gas in their stomach

2. "I've become a little older since I saw you last," says one friend to another, "and a few changes have come into my life. Frankly, I've become quite a frivolous gal—I'm seeing five gentlemen at the same time.

"As soon as I wake up, Will Power helps me out of bed. Then I go to John. Then Charlie Horse comes along, and he takes a lot of my time and attention. After he leaves, Arthur Ritis shows up and stays with me for the rest of the day. He doesn't want to stay in one place for too long, so he takes me from joint to joint. After such a busy day, I'm really tired and glad when I can go to bed with Ben Gay.

"Oh what a life!"

3. The preacher came a-calling the other day. He said at my age I ought to think about the hereafter. "But I do that all the time," I assured him. "No matter where I am, in the basement, the kitchen or the attic, I always ask myself: What am I here after?"

Yes, Jane liked to laugh. But for us, you and I, it's time to get serious again. I'll just add a word right quick about acupuncture. I'm a little afraid of the thought of having needles… (No, I ain't saying "I'd never…" I had to eat those words too often. Another example of my having changed my stubborn mind once again is below.)

MSWGMD

For years, two of my sisters-in-law swore they had been helped by chiropractors. I triple-harrumphed at that, and sometimes used pretty strong denigrating language to voice my rejection of the field, up to 1990 or thereabouts.

My husband had succeeded into nagging, cajoling and bribing me into keeping the appointment he had made for me at a chiropractic clinic. Reluctantly, grumbling and inwardly swearing it would do me no good, even once or twice vociferously objecting, we arrived at the clinic. Of course we had to wait. I hung on to my ugliest face and would have marched off if I hadn't been called at that very moment.

In the doorway of the office stood the doctor, a slender, fragile-looking and soft-spoken lady. She welcomed me, took my medical history, looked at the X-rays I had brought along, confirmed the arthritis in neck, knee and ankles and didn't say a word, didn't even look disapproving at my admission of smoking and proclaiming my intention of not planning to stop.

But what impressed me the most was her factualness, her making neither claims nor promises, just kindly saying she'd try to help me as much as she could.

And, ladies and gentlemen, help me she did! Many times since that first reluctant visit. Alleviated the stiffness in neck, back and hip, the sinus pains, the TMJ-jaw pains, even the excruciating pain of a pulled sciatic nerve. Now whenever I'm in pain or get stiffish, I call on her and her expertise.

Oh, and after my son injured his back in 1997 in a car accident and muscle relaxers and pain pills didn't grant him adequate relief, he made an appointment with my chiropractor's husband, practicing in the same clinic. My daughter attended several sessions in 1999 and received relief from her discomforts. Now her husband has horrible back pains, and she said Sunday that she'll make an appointment for him to go there.

The moral of that mind-change of another of my "I'll never...": One should keep an open mind, have the courage to admit one had drawn a wrong conclusion and changed said mind. (I have admitted so far to several of those mind-changes, huh.)

MSWGMD

The next item came to me via three sources—my son, our CR and my chiropractor—and it still leaves me looking around, expecting the famous buzzing.

The article sent by our CR told, in word and pictures, the story of Pat Wagner who let herself be stung 5,000 times and said with each sting she felt better, more energetic and her vision improved.

My chiropractor sent me *Alternatives for the Health Conscious Individual*. It carried an article that stated that bee venom therapy can deliver great benefits, not only for persons with MS, but also for those who suffer from other inflammatory conditions. (One of those, I suppose, could be arthritis.) The author also talked about research on bee venom going on, especially in Europe and Japan.

Well, finally the National jumped on the bandwagon and awarded a grant to study the effects of bee venom on MS.

Update for 2002: It has finally caught on in the States too and aggressive research has been started here.

My son sent me the cover story of "Neighborhood Times" which is a twice-weekly supplement to the *St. Petersburg Times*. It carried a lengthy story about a beehive being moved so that a woman with MS could "use the bees in her therapy for multiple sclerosis." She asserted that twenty bee stings per day kept her free of MS symptoms.

Hm, well, I do like to feel better, but I'm kinda glad I have the legitimate excuse of being highly allergic to bee stings. I'd rather wait till they come up with something I can take by mouth or inject.

MSWGMD

Now a few items about dietary therapies. They all come from copies my chiropractor had made for me. I neither endorse nor reject either one of them but offer them for consideration to anybody who may be interested.

The magazine *Health Counselor* (16-20 April 1996) carried the story of an MS person who had changed her diet to no salt, no sugar, no friend food, no red meat. She drank a lot of vegetable and fruit juices. Her MS, as of this 1996 writing, was in total remission; she worked full time and felt great. Her conclusion: Diet can alleviate many multiple sclerosis symptoms.

Another *Health Counselor* reported on Dr. Christine Neuhofer. She is an MSer herself and advocates enzyme therapy as disease-fighters. She uses an enzyme mixture and achieved dramatic results for herself and two hundred MS persons whom she had treated.

Incidentally, this issue estimated the number of people afflicted with MS as 500,000.

MSWGMD

The mother of another young man who was diagnosed as having MS sent me an article and a note. The article talked about a fourteen-year-old boy stricken with ALD (adrenoleukodystrophy). The movie *Lorenzo's Oil* told the story of this young man's and his parents' brave struggles. I finally got to see the movie and found it quite good. Our CR was intrigued by it too and saw MS-implications.

As I understand it, ALD is a rare, genetic, demyelinating disease, and the search for a cure runs along similar lines as the search for a cure for MS. But the over-cautious medical director of the National would not cooperate. I will reprint part of that lady's comments; she sums it up beautifully:

> …We were a little upset with the doctor's comments about not cooperating in research that clearly is of benefit to multiple sclerosis and for commenting that research should

not progress too rapidly. Do we need to waste another generation of patients to satisfy his time table?

(I don't know if that gentleman is still with the National or not.)

I did receive Public Affairs Department News Memo 8-93 (dated February 6, 1993). It said that Croda Universal Ltd, Hull, England, is developing a dietary supplement oil to be tested as a treatment for multiple sclerosis because it has been found that certain oils are missing in MS patients. This is the company which manufactured Lorenzo's Oil.

I have not heard or seen any more about this.

During the updating process, something hit me. You remember my remark about scientists jealously guarding their research results to be the first who can proclaim the success of the discovery? I also spoke of the fact that I as well as others believe the National sponsors research which will confirm their theories? Maybe this medical director wanted to protect the research of the National's grantees? Or maybe through not sharing the gleaned info they can shout: "I'm the first who..."

Oh, I don't know; maybe I'm rambling. Will you join me in that? Maybe we can come up with something we can rub their noses in to speed the process up?   .

MSWGMD

On July 28, 1996, new uses for the old drug Thalidomide was featured on the CBS program *60 Minutes*. Leslie Stahl was the reporter. She began by showing the usual pictures about the horror of children and adults who had been born disfigured after their mothers had taken the drug. The rest of the report though was different. Ms. Stahl said that Thalidomide is being re-researched, that it can work on the immune system, is being considered as treatment for AIDS, tuberculosis, some cancers, rheumatoid arthritis and lupus. Finally she specifically mentioned that it may be helpful to multiple sclerosis patients.

Of course some people objected to it being revived, but I mean, come on, men don't get pregnant, and women who are past child-bearing age or had a hysterectomy can't incur the potential of bearing damaged children.

But the bottom line was that people can be helped and that some in that report had asserted they had obtained great relief.

Update: I have read that Thalidomide has already proved its worth, although I didn't see whether it has been prescribed for people with MS.

MSWGMD

The Winter 1993 *MS Relay* printed revised numbers of MS cases in the US. I had previously complained many times that the number of MS cases steadily stood at 250,000. A while ago, they upped it to 350,000. In that 1993 *Relay* issue, they finally said the numbers were around 450,000. (Remember, you read a few pages ago that others said the numbers of MS cases in the US are as high as 500,000 and, according to Montel Williams, may be as high as 1.8 million.) I wonder what the correct numbers for almost-2005 are.

I have read the estimate that about two hundred people are being diagnosed with MS each week. But in 2002, it was back down to 350,000. I ask you: How? Why? MSers aren't cured, and MS doesn't shorten the normal life span.

I don't know who sets these numbers, gives them out as facts and who benefits from keeping the estimates artificially low, whether it's the National or the NIH, (the National Institute of Health) or whomever, but the 450,000 to 500,00 sound a bit more realistic to me.

Symptoms

In the 1990s, our group members were interested in hearing what the lesions in specific parts of the brain were doing to specific parts of the MSer's body; that is, which symptoms they cause. I have updated that material too. If you want to refresh your memory on where specific brain areas are located and what their major functions are, remember some of that is explained in the Brain Definitions section.

Brainstem-Cerebellar Lesions: For as small as that area is, brainstem-cerebellar lesions bring on quite a few nasty problems. Beginning with the eyes, these lesions cause double vision, blurred vision, involuntary movement of the eyeball, inability to focus, blind spots in the vision field and loss of peripheral vision.

Other problems blameable on brainstem-cerebellum lesions: In union with other brain areas, they bring on the trouble with coordination and balance—the gait and ataxia problems. Also, difficulty with chewing, swallowing and hampered communication through slurred speech. Add the tremors when trying to reach for something, the darned and infamous clumsiness.

I have not read or heard this as a fact, but I would wager a guess that the vertigo also stems from lesions in this area.

Spinal Cord Lesions: Demyelination there bring some doozies of symptoms. When the below-the-neck area is affected, a person can expect the pins-and-needles sensation; the limbs—arms and/or legs—feel numb; movements are clumsy; skin feels cold. There can be pain, which feels as if an electric shock courses through one's body. (Remember, I call that insect bites on the inside of my body.)

If you have these spinal cord lesions, you may complain about an arm or leg feeling heavy or weak or just not working right. In other words, if it affects the arm, you can't lift the coffee cup, let alone the whole pot. If it affects the leg or legs, you have trouble putting one foot in front of the other, which, to say the least, makes walking, running and climbing stairs difficult. (The limb feeling rigid or stiff is a sign of spasticity.)

There are other difficulties layable on the spinal cord:

Bowel, bladder and sexual problems go to it. We can't feel it when a finger or toe is moved slightly or when the skin is touched gently. Not to forget being unable to handle small objects—sewing needles, paper clips, buttons. Oh, the spinal cord gangs up with other brain areas, and they combine to cause the unsteadiness and stumbling around.

MSWGMD

It is being said that cerebrum-caused disabilities come later in the course of the disease and are clustered around the term "intellectual dysfunctions." (The National had one or two great Facts & Issues reports on that subject available. I'm sure it's still available.)

I have heard there may be a lot of lesions in the cerebrum (the neocortex), but by 1996, they had not been mapped out completely yet. So on the morning of March 28, 2002, I spent about two hours on the Internet. I received confirmation of the facts I have presented above. (Please recall what I said about the involvement of the gray matter in the iron deposits entry.) It also said I was right in my conjecture that vertigo stems from brainstem-cerebellum lesions. But I could not find a thing about neocortex lesions or lesions in the limbic system and what symptoms they cause.

It is odd, as much knowledge as the brain has released of some of its wonders, it still is the undiscovered mystery frontier, wide open for exploration. It has not been mapped out as the genome project has done for the genetics field. We still know only bits and pieces, which need to be fitted together eventually.

For myself, though, I took time out to look at the lobes of the cerebral hemispheres, compared them with my symptoms and pinpointed roughly where the lesions were hidden. The MRI later proved that I had been basically correct.

MSWGMD

Talking about vertigo though. I had severe, even incapacitating bouts of it, couldn't see right, couldn't read, couldn't see the TV pictures and needed the walker instead of just the cane to move about without falling. At my last visit with the neurologist I mentioned it and two days later they called me so set up a consult with another doctor. (I'm sorry, I still don't know her specialty but I know she was connected with the neurology department.) She put me through one and a half hours of non-invasive tests which reminded me somewhat of the evoked responses tests. It surprised me though to notice that most tests were concentrating on the eyes instead of the ear or specifically the middle ear.

At the completion, she said that she had good and bad news. The bad news was that it was my left side that gave me problems, and I affirmed that as being the MS-affected side. The good news was that something could be done—it being a repositioning procedure. I got an appointment for the following Friday, underwent a couple of non-invasive procedures, had to wear a neck brace for forty-eight hours and haven't been bothered by vertigo since then.

It must be something new because at my next neuro appointment, the nurse quizzed me about it extensively because, she said, I had been the first one who had gone through the complete procedure. Even as I called for my July 2004 appointment, she waned to know about this procedure.

Well, all I can say is, "Thank God, it worked."

MSWGMD

Words of warning though—and please don't forget them.

People who have MS are not immune to other illnesses. Like ordinary people, we get colds, sore throats and laryngitis. We're hit with cancers, ulcers and arteriosclerosis. Osteo- and rheumatoid arthritis or diabetes doesn't pass us by just because we have MS. Our eyes are not only affected by optic neuritis, but we're also far- or near-sighted, have astigmatism, get cataracts. A host of smaller or larger aches and pains come our way and should be checked out by the family doctor.

In other words, don't deceive yourself and blame everything on the poor MS; check things out with your family doctor. At least see him or her occasionally.

Now I know I ought to take my own advice—at least occasionally—but outside of the MS and the arthritis, I'm quite healthy, am helped by my chiropractor and otherwise doctor myself with over-the-counter medications. I did have to have complete physical exams before I could schedule my cataract surgery. (Yeah, my ophthalmologist insisted on it because it's the law in Ohio. He refused to take my word that I was in perfect health—which was proved by the tests.) Otherwise, I never had a broken bone; my only hospital stays were at age nine to have my appendix removed, then at age fourteen, the tonsils came out, and between twenty-four and thirty, I had my kids. The first stitches I had at age fifty-one after I cut myself on a glass in the dishwashing water.

Yes, I know I am blessed.

MSWGMD

I want to end this segment with an interesting fact as food for thought. In the book *Living with Multiple Sclerosis* by Marcella Z. Davis is a sentence worth perusing. It says that doctors are not sure whether the MS symptoms stem from stress or from the plagues. (I just wanted to draw your attention to it. Uh, sorry, sometimes I can't help myself but rub against those who talk theory instead of those who experience it.)

Some News from Galion, Ohio

Note: The following facts and data are unrevised numbers from 1996. Since I have retired from the support group and it suspended operation, I am not privy to the newest information any longer.

Those of you who receive the magazine *Inside MS* for some time may have read the article in the Summer 1989 issue titled "Researching Clusters," which mentioned our town, population 12,391 at that time.

Following is a summary of facts from an active participant and observer of the study. In 1982, Galion had an apparently unusual high number of people diagnosed as having multiple sclerosis. The then-Deputy Health Commissioner (a wonderful lady, even if we disagreed strongly on seatbelts and smoking) and two concerned Galionites discussed that and persuaded the Ohio Department of Health (ODH) to investigate those incidents. One of the ladies was the mother of a young man who had MS and later died (the same one who brought us the mercury in teeth information and otherwise was a great benefactor of our group); the other lady had MS herself and became the founder and first president of the local MS support group.

The ODH's team conducted extensive written and verbal interviews, did blood work, interviewed physicians and compared MS cases with appropriate non-MS controls of similar age, gender, occupation and length of residence in Galion, one MS person being contrasted with four controls.

By the time the study results came in, I had joined the support group, had been appointed secretary and soon added public relations, research and newsletter writing to my duties. The ODH issued a report on this study and determined that as of March 8, 1990, there lived eighteen persons with a legitimate MS diagnosis in Galion and Polk Township. On June 24, 1990, the Galion Deputy Health Commissioner and the Chief of the Division of Epidemiology from the ODH briefed the Crawford Multiple Sclerosis Support Group members and representatives of the media on the results of the study.

Our local newspaper, the *Galion Inquirer*, printed a detailed report of the meeting. (I
needed it.)

Along with the findings, the ODH's Division Chief also recommended that "the prevalence of MS in Galion be recalculated...(yearly) to determine whether the high
observed prevalence of MS changes over time and at what rate." (Please keep that in mind; I will return to it momentarily.)

ODH's Summary and Conclusions

Number two of the Report's Conclusions: The case-control studies identified several factors as associated with the disease: "Higher educational attainment." From the summary: "Cases...graduated from high school (most not in Galion) and from college. This is a well-known feature of MS from other studies."

Continuing from the Report's Conclusions: "...having received oral polio vaccine, a history of allergies, having one or more relatives with a neurological disease and having a cat that died from unexplained causes were all significantly higher in cases than in controls. Cases also had slightly higher titers of HTLV-1, the Human T-Cell Lymphotropic Virus-1, than controls, but this difference was not statistically significant. [You recall my write-up under Research.] Cases did not differ from controls in blood levels of lead, mercury, arsenic and cadmium."

Personal Addendum: In other words, they did not find anything specific—did not find the expected environmental trigger—to account for the higher-than-normal rate of MS incidents in Galion at the time, considering the numbers of people they had to work with.

As regards to educational attainment, it is not vainglorious self-glorification, but MS tends to strike smart people, and that's a fact documented in several studies and catalogued in written literature.

What do you think about that? I admit I still puzzle over it without finding anything that makes sense, except that maybe we use our brains more?

Regarding HTLV-1, the Report cited "statistically not significant levels" showing up. Well, I say, if it's in there (in our bodies, I mean), it should be investigated or the results forwarded to appropriate researchers who investigate this specific field of MS.

You also notice that one of the first Conclusions stated "having one or more relatives who had a neurological disease." Now if that shows up among our small numbers, how does it relate to the totality of the MS population nationwide?

Many Galionites were surprised, and some disappointed because ODH didn't find more heavy metals residue in the cases. Those who initiated the study to begin with were convinced of something being in soil, water or air to cause these excessive numbers of MS cases in our city. But the tests said no.

Okay, that remark in regards to me needing the newspaper article? Well, you see, during that meeting, I sat next to a young man (my daughter swore he had a crush on me, but I had never noticed). Instead of dutifully taking the copious notes I was supposed to take to prepare an intelligent report for the newsletter and a write-up for the *Galion Inquirer*'s Meeting Briefs, I had whispered and exchanged cut-ups with him.

Well, due to my inattentiveness toward the speakers and the empty pages in my notebook, I had to educate myself on that newspaper article the next day to post a halfway decent report for the Meeting Briefs. Thank goodness I received the detailed report from the ODH before the next newsletter was due.

But dang it, it sure was a fun meeting for us two.

P.S. to that: I still am grateful to *Galion Inquirer* reporter Eric Smith, who did such an excellent job on general and specific MS reportings.

MSWGMD

That article in *Inside MS* I spoke about in the beginning, it talked about a study performed by the Cleveland (Ohio) Clinic. The findings of that study were, in my opinion, uh, not quite factual. You can't imagine what sorts of adverbs and adjectives floated through my mind, so I'll just say that many conclusions were erroneous, drawn superficially, not considering all the facts. Actually, some people insisted it smelled to them as if the Cleveland Clinic wanted to upstage the ODH. We in Galion did not give much credibility to that study, especially since not all who participated in the ODH study trekked to Cleveland. (I for one did not. And, uhuh, the ODH came to Galion to deal courteously with us. The health nurse came to the MSers' house to take the blood samples and talk to the individual people one on one. The Cleveland Clinic made people drive up there, and the few who went complained bitterly about the impersonal treatment, the long waits and not "being told anything."

MSWGMD

Okay, a moment ago I requested you hold a thought about recalculating the rate of MS prevalence in Galion. Here is why:

In 1992, an epidemiologist from the ODH contacted me, and we mapped out a plan on how to go about getting her the facts for the follow-up study without my breaking the seal of confidentiality.

I notified the Chapter, and they shut me down. I re-contacted them, explained in detail, verbally and in writing what I had arranged, but for months, nothing happened. I decided finally that I had waited long enough. I consulted with the other two officers; they granted approval of my plan; I initiated actions, handed chairperson and treasurer their letters, filled out mine and sent out twenty-seven explanatory letters to people known to be diagnosed with multiple sclerosis. Included in the letter of explanation was a pre-addressed, stamped postcard, requesting permission to forward the person's name to the ODH. In the letter I outlined what I needed, numbered each item and only wrote the numbers "1" and "2" on the card, the pertinent data to be filled in by the MS person.

The cards trickled back in, but despite several requests via mail, a plea in the *Galion Inquirer* and two notes in the newsletter, only nineteen people responded. (That included us three officers.) Finally I had to concede defeat and forwarded what I had permission to forward. The results disappointed me, the ODH, the Galion Deputy Health Commissioner, the people from the support group and concerned Galionites, but what could the ODH do? They could not unprofessionally work with unsubstantiated data just relying on my word of it being so, and an increase of only four cases in almost two years did not indicate a major rise in the Galion MS population.

MSWGMD

Following are the true facts as of February 14, 1993:

Including us officers, we had the names of thirty people with a firm and confirmed MS diagnosis on our mailing list, and they had physically resided in Galion proper during the time of the on-going study. That included the eight who had not responded to the permission request. Five people with an MS diagnosis had died during the period, and three had moved very recently. We knew of at least five more people living in Galion who had been diagnosed but had chosen not to come forward and be counted.

This makes forty-three recognized cases who had lived in Galion during the intervening time of the study's initial testings and the follow-up. If that doesn't qualify our small city to be named a cluster city, I don't know who would or should or could.

I want to beg here: If you are being asked to be counted, please respond. There is strength in numbers. If the block of MS persons increases, our ranking increases, and we qualify for more research time and money.

MSWGMD

A few more facts came to my attention during the time I was involved with this study: These are all verifiable facts.

1. Three males were born within eighteen months of each other, in close proximity in Galion. All three developed MS and died within eighteen months of each other.

2. The little town of Crestline, Ohio, just a few miles away from Galion, population approximately 5,000, had eight MS cases that we knew of. Nobody, including me, would be surprised if there had not been a few more. In fact, toward the end of 2002, my daughter's best friend, a young lady I consider my "second daughter," was diagnosed with multiple sclerosis. Up to her marriage about seven or eight years ago, she lived here in Galion and then moved to Crestline.

3. Three people of approximately the same age (not the three males cited in number 1 above) lived on three street corners in Crestline, and all three developed MS. One of them was our treasurer, a second one was also a member of our support group, and I know the third person. They all assured me that this was the truth.

4. The age of MSers I know ranges from the early twenty to the late sixties.

5. Several people, who gave up the fight, developed severe exacerbations and died.

Chapter Five
Help and Helpers

There are the National and the Chapter (mentioned earlier), other organizations and gadgets (mentioned shortly), but the best help, in my opinion, is a good locally managed support group.

I have heard many objections to joining one.

"Somebody might recognize me, and I don't want anybody to know."

"They're probably just a bunch of crybabies who feel sorry for themselves and exchange sobsister stories. I don't need that."

"They're probably just a mutual admiration club."

"They're probably in worse shape than I am, and I don't want to see what might happen to me in the future."

"I'm probably in better shape than they are, and I'd feel guilty about that or they'd resent me."

Well, let me talk about our support group, what we did, how we did it, how we helped each other. Also, in case you belong to a support group and are dissatisfied or in case you want to start one, maybe the following can give you some tips on how to go about it.

These are my visions of what a support group could be, what it could do and how it could help:

At your support group,

    * you can ask questions and find info, help, encouragement and inspiration.

    * you can gripe and know listeners will understand what you're talking about because they go through similar difficulties, fear similar fears, experience similar positive or negative emotions.

    * you find a shoulder to cry on and know that at the same place you find the strongest bunch of people who will help you up again when you feel down.

    * you find people who cope with their disabilities, can make fun of them and the limitation they encounter.

    * you can share your trials, fears and tribulations as well as your triumphs, successes and victories.

    * you can mingle with people who bravely face up to carrying the burdens they have been loaded down with, make the best of it and help others carry their millstone

    * you don't need to feel intimidated by your disability, need not fear somebody could think of you as damaged merchandise or see you as an invalid.

And isn't that something worth creating, attending and participating in?

MSWGMD

I had written the following for our group, presented it to the Chapter, and they adopted it as official literature to be distributed throughout their service area. The then-Chapter Services Director worked hard to make it an attractive little brochure. I want to reprint it here for you. (Yes, I'm darn proud of it.) Incidentally, we had that conversation about MSers not being patients during work on this brochure.

She titled it:

> Others who know...
> Others who care...

What Is a Multiple Sclerosis Support Group

Multiple sclerosis—a word that fills people with a multitude of negative emotions. Not many people know much about the disease, but particularly here in northern Ohio, nearly everybody knows someone with MS.

A lot of confusion surrounds multiple sclerosis because it affects every patient differently. No two patients share the same symptoms, complaints or course of illness. "MS is as individual as the individual people affected with it," a neurologist said once in answer to a patient's question.

Multiple sclerosis is difficult to diagnose, the diagnosis is difficult to accept, and life as an MS person is sometimes difficult because the only sure thing about multiple sclerosis is its unpredictability.

But There Is Hope

Hope is needed to face up to and cope with multiple sclerosis, and some of this hope is dispensed by the members of the Multiple Sclerosis Support Group. We at the Support Group are here

* to prove to persons newly diagnosed with MS that there is life after an MS diagnosis.

* to help those searching for information to find out as much as possible or suggest sources where answers can be found.

* to cheer on our members in remission and hope it will stay so forever.

* to show worried members who are in the midst of an exacerbation that they are not alone.

* to show the angry MS person that it is all right to be angry and that anger is not a bad emotion that nice people shouldn't have.

* for members who want to talk, someone is always within reach by phone or mail.

* to convince those who doubt their worth as human beings that they still are as worthy individuals as they were before they were diagnosed as having MS.

* for people who believe their lives now lack worth, value and meaning: we tell them in the support group meetings (once a month) through our newsletter (bi-monthly) on the phone or by mail (anytime), "Don't despair. Don't get permanently discouraged. Don't ever give up hope, no matter how bad MS treats you. You are still important. You still contribute to family, friends and society. You still count."

* to disprove the self-doubting MS person or the unkind thoughtlessness of people who believe having MS is a disgrace or cause for guilt and shame or that MS is a punishment for something bad they have done.

* for the family members or friends of MS persons who wonder what their loved ones go through, where they can go to talk to someone and how they can help each other.

In the words of one of our support group member:

Yes, there is hope
And hope for a cure
At the end of the rainbow

Our Crawford MS Support Group

Note: Please remember: I don't want to brag about our group. I just want to give you an inkling of what we did and how we did it. Maybe it will inspire you to start a group, become actively involved in one or revive a mired-down one.

I wanted to begin with "Our support group came into bloom in 1988," but I believe I have to start a bit farther back because—and I'm proud of that too—I helped it to take shape.

As I said earlier, I was diagnosed in 1982 and had just overcome the "MS having me" attitude. Thus in 1987, I was ready to attended a meeting of MS persons, their families and interested community members. They discussed the formation of an MS support group, but I didn't feel like attending the first three or four regular meetings. In April 1988, the first chairman of the group called me and hit me over the head with the declaration: "You're gonna write our newsletters for us. I'll bring the stuff over in a little while, okay?" She did come, dumped a folder and a few pieces of handwritten material and some paper on my table, and didn't listen to my plea that I had no idea how to do a newsletter. She reminded me of the work I had done at the school and asked me come to the next meeting. She said I'd get enough material to fill the pages. After saying all that, she patted me on the shoulder and left.

Hm, becoming an active member and attend the support group meetings? I had never officially belonged to a group except being the leader of a Catholic girls' youth group in my early twenties and attending a few meetings at the US Army's Officers' Wives Club in the seventies, and as I'd wailed, I didn't have the faintest idea of how to write a newsletter.

But, as I said in the foreword, I'd give it one heck of a try, and of course I picked up the technique. I attended the meeting in April 1988, put the first newsletter together, and, *boing*, everything—my life, my outlook on people and my attitude toward MS—changed.

Over the summer of 1988, the group underwent changes in format, structure and leadership. In September, I received my first appointment as secretary and newsletter editor and also took over the public relations; that is, announcing regular meetings and special events to the public, writing post-meeting notices and speaking publicly in schools, nursing homes and on TV to promote MS awareness.

Let me tell you, it was lots of work, but I loved every minute of it. Normally I reserve the word "love" for special people and use "like" for things, but working with the group and for the group, I loved doing.

As I said, I had never been a member of a group; thus I had no idea on how to do officering either, but I learned. I suppose that happens in a labor of love.

The Meetings

We met once monthly, keeping those get-togethers totally informal, and didn't charge any dues. Sometimes we had speakers, as you saw in the "What They Said" section; at other times, we had open forums where we concentrated on discussing one specific subject. The open gabfests usually turned out the best and were the most satisfying; in addition, they allowed us to get to know each other better. That, and being a small group, helped in building trust; we could be honest with each other about our thoughts and feelings, and through that, we gave others permission to be honest about themselves, their thoughts and feelings too.

In January, to lighten up the winter doldrums, we had our Christmas-in-January party, with raffles, door prizes, good food, good talk and lots of laughter.

In August, we held our picnic/major fundraiser with, well, see above, with the other attraction being the water balloon fights.

At first I didn't notice any one-upmanship or backstabbing, but in the final months of my tenure as an officer these negativities raised their ugly heads so severely that even I could no longer fail to notice them—and that hurt. But I am sure that neither of us three officers felt uppity toward the general membership; we were only responsible for putting the programs together, took care of the paperwork and the money, and acted as go-betweens of Chapter, community and group.

What We Officers Did

Before the 1991 election, I told the group members what each of us three officers did and asked who wanted to become more actively involved in running the group, to either take on a full or partial position.

Here is the outline of what I said. This basic structure didn't change much through three top leadership changes.

We three officers—president, treasurer and secretary—gathered one week before the meeting and discussed the business which had accumulated over the past weeks and inform the others of what we had done for the group. Then we planned and outlined the meeting. Having become friends over the years of working for the good of the group, we also shared personal concerns or gripes which were too delicate to be aired in group.

I don't want to spook potential candidates, but here is what we do: Our president (two of them, preferred to be called chairperson) is responsible for the overall running of the group. She takes care of the paperwork and brings our complaints and concerns to the proper channels to get the best deal for us. She also lines up speakers and holds the reins at the meetings.

At this point, I thanked the outgoing leader and proceeded to the treasurer's position.

Our treasurer takes care of the money, which comes in and goes out of course, but she does so much more. She writes the greeting cards for birthdays and anniversaries, the get-well and sympathy cards and thank you notes. She is also in charge of the raffles; along with her husband, she puts the summer picnic together and takes care of the books in the lending library and the literature from the Chapter. She also calls ahead to make sure the church door is open at six o'clock each second Tuesday of the month.

I thanked her and her husband and then proceeded to the toughest part—talking about myself and what I did.

I'm the secretary, take care of the correspondence, the announcements of the meetings in the three area newspapers, the radio and the TV station. After the meeting, I write up summary notices for the "Meeting Briefs" in the area's newspapers.

I'm also the psychology nut in residence; being a bookworm, I'm in charge of research. Every two months, I put together and type up the newsletter. After it is printed, I ready it for mailing.

Otherwise I do everything I can to make people aware of the existence of our group and show what we can do to help anybody who has multiple sclerosis or is concerned about a person who has multiple sclerosis.

That ended my speech, and expectantly, I looked around. I received a polite round of applause; one of the group members said, since we had done such a good job, we should be held over for another year. Before she had finished, other members piped in with "I second that," and we were in for another year. Incidentally, the same thing happened in 1992 and 1993. That is, the treasurer and I stayed for the full five years; the president/chairperson position changed hands or imaginary-gavels three times. (It changed a fourth time after I resigned.)

The Newsletter

Note: Please remember; I don't want to fill pages, but I believe each of these reprinted introductions carries a message, and I hope they can help you and inspire you to not ever consider giving up. At least not longer than an hour or so.

It came out every second month; later on, I could write it monthly or more when I had something special to announce. The following shows what I wrote in newsletter #1. I introduced myself and my purpose and wrote the following:

> I would like to make this your newsletter, writing what you contribute, giving you some thoughts that will help you between the group's meetings, showing you that you are not alone, add a few words that might give you some comfort and encouragement and show you that you are not alone but are one of a darn tough and strong bunch of people who won't give MS the satisfaction of having defeated us.
>
> Tell us about your joys and pleasures, and let us be happy with you. Talking about your concerns could bring about our helping you through offering suggestions for solutions. Sharing your trials and tribulations, as well as how you overcome or overcame and deal with them, could be helpful to others. For instance, you could tell us about your ideas, tips and hints on how you cope with life, health and illness. You could recommend a book you found helpful, interesting or simply well-written, could warn us about another one that isn't worth wasting our time or tell us about a good movie. A joke would brighten somebody's day and take away the gloominess.

Also helpful item would be "Point of View," "How I Do It," or "Food for Thought" pieces. All that could show others that they are not alone or give them hope, a new outlook or viewpoint.

In short, let's share anything that comes to your mind, something you find worthwhile, something that might help somebody else overcome times of doubt and fear.

Would you be interested in a telephone support line? We could make this—the support group, the newsletter and the phone line—the Fearsome Threesome that chases the MS blues away.

This Fearsome Threesome would consist of people who endure similar difficulties. Sure, we are all individualistic individuals with distinctively different MS complaints, but at least sometimes we are all weighed down, and from time to time we are overwhelmed by depression, sadness, even despair. We all feel lonely at times and wish we could speak with somebody who would understand us; we go through our specific triumphs and terrors, face hopes and fears, have to work through acceptance and anger problems and have to muster the strength to overcome weakness of body, mind, soul and spirit.

I say we can make life easier for ourselves and others, so let's band together and be there for each other, to talk, to encourage, to give sympathy and understanding born out of empathy.

So won't you please jot down your thoughts, questions and suggestions, bring them to the meeting, send them to…or call…

MSWGMD

Sounded good, didn't it? (At least I thought so.) I'm sorry to report thought that nothing came of it. We officers received an occasional phone call; I received an occasional praise for what I had said in the newsletter; the number of people attending the meetings stayed steadily at twelve to eighteen; the former chairperson and the treasurer contributed an occasional write-up or poem; our CR faithfully contributed the news clippings she found and added her personal notations. A later plea in April 1992 didn't produce anything either.

Yes, I was a little sad but accepted it. I kept eyes and ears open for anything of interest and continued to write the newsletter for the five years that I was associated with the group.

MSWGMD

Now some specifics. The Chapter had sent us some material with the heading of HOPE. I begged them to let me use it as the heading for my newsletter, and since the two pieces of literature were completely different, I received the permission.

Beside that logo, I typed the names and phone numbers of our officers; beneath that came a dedication to special people who deserved recognition—spouses, children, friends, benefactors of the group, the lady at the *Galion Inquirer* who put my informal language into printable copy—just anybody who, as I said, deserved a special thank you or recognition. (I had to conserve space since I had only two legal-size or three regular-size pages available to mail it with the then-twenty-nine cent first-class stamp.)

I began the single-spaced body of the newsletter with "Hi, Everybody," followed by a short introduction (a few samples shortly), a description of the last meeting, news from the MS world, an occasional book report or whatever I came up with. Usually I had to end on short notice because I had more to write than I had space for. I ended—and still use that phrase in most of my correspondence or on the MS bulletin boards—with "Best wishes for permanent remission. Elvie."

MSWGMD

As fundraisers and to keep our financial independence from the Chapter, to pay for paper, postage stamps and other incidentals, we raffled off items which had been donated-a little plant, a coffee cup, a bowl-at the end of our meetings. During the summer picnic/fundraiser we raffled off items our treasurer had scrounged up or anything somebody had donated. A few of us collected aluminum cans, and our treasurer's husband sold them for us. We received occasional cash contributions, and when necessary—let's say to buy meat, paper plates and plastic ware for the Christmas-in-January party—we could turn to the Chapter for financial assistance.

MSWGMD

After our corps of officer took over, we, with the best of intentions, planned an enthusiastic recruiting program. After all, we had a good program to offer that could help somebody carry their heavy load; maybe we could even lighten it a bit. All we needed to do was getting our message out. The *Galion Inquirer* helped us, and the local TV station invited us to do a half-hour program, which our treasurer and I attended. We got all the names we could get our hands on and got ready to call the people on our lists.

Well, I called the chapter services director and proudly informed her of our intentions, but she said: "Whoa, hold it. You can't do that. Some people don't want to belong to a support group."

"That's okay," I confidently shot back. "We only want to call them, let them know about us, and then they can come to the meetings, ask to be put on the mailing list only, ask for other info or simply ignore us."

Well, the lady didn't tell me to shut up and listen; she explained patiently that some people don't want anybody to know that they have MS, not even their families. Because so little is known about the illness and because so much disinformation, so many myths and scares are spouted forth, people hide the fact that they are stricken with it. Employers could get spooked; insurance companies could drop the one with a chronic disease; strangers, acquaintances, friends, even family members could retreat in horror and fear of catching it. (I think now that it is simply the fear of the unknown.)

Well, that was one of the few times I was miffed at her. We officers called her "overcautious." Uh, well, we did use unkinder terms and really grumbled. After some hindsight-thinking though, I realized she had been more than right, and I, in my enthusiasm, had gone overboard.

I just had to look a myself. How long had I kept it a secret that I had MS? And having worked in a Drug and Alcohol Assistance Center, I should have recalled the master lesson I had been inculcated with, the lesson of keeping confidentialities confidential, first, last and always. (Different people had tried all sorts of tricks to make me reveal who was in the program, but, I'm proud to say, nobody ever caught me off-guard.) In the next newsletter, I admitted to my thoughtlessness and assured our support group members and the newsletter readers of the same respect in safeguarding their names and anything else entrusted to me. Also, anything with a name on it, plus the list of recipients of the newsletter, was kept in my locked briefcase.

From then on, I used every precaution possible. I never used names in the newspaper write-ups or the newsletters. I never gave out names, addresses or phone numbers unless I had obtained permission to do so first. I was familiar with most of the families of the regulars; I'm sure they recognized my German accent, and I knew when I could talk openly. When I phoned someone whose family circumstances I was not familiar with, I left my name and phone number and said something to the effect that I had a message I was supposed to deliver, but not the reason why I was calling or with what organization I was affiliated. For instance, as I mentioned earlier, we knew of at least five people who were diagnosed as having multiple sclerosis and would have liked to offer them our assistance, but because they had not contacted us, we had to leave them alone.

But one thing I did do. I wrote an open letter to hospitals, rehabilitation and physical therapy services, as well as the offices of neurologists that I knew were frequented by area MS persons. I requested they direct MS persons to a letter of introduction from us. You find a copy of what I wrote in the Appendix.

We three officers tried in other ways to make people aware of our existence. We participated in a parade, but couldn't wave because we couldn't stop laughing and had to hide it. We participated in a health fair. The Galion Health Department, the public library and word of mouth directed people to us. The mailing list for the newsletter grew from thirty-three to eighty-seven, and the phone calls for information came more frequent. We were established as a viable group in the community.

Being an Officer

Basically we had fun in our group, did a lot of laughing and talking, sharing and learning. But no, it wasn't all fun and games for us officers. We had our frustrations, disagreements and misunderstandings. Feelings got hurt. One didn't like what the other did or said. The delicate balance between Chapter and group got strained. The members' consumer-type taking what we offered, their apathy and non-participation hurt, even irritated and aggravated.

And yes, although we were very enthusiastic about our group, we officers got burned out from giving and caring and doing. After all, we were just normal, imperfect human beings.

(My kids call me too idealistic—expecting too much of people and not seeing the bad things—but I tell them, that's me; it's one aspect of my personality, and I can't do much about it. In fact, I don't want to do much about it.)

A question: When you are an officer and are depressed, frightened, in the dumps, need somebody to hold you up, where do you go?

I was blessed with my friendship with Jane, our treasurer. She and I were honest with each other, but basically, I'm afraid most of the time you'll deal with it by yourself. You don't want to bother the other officers because you think it's your responsibility to put up the good front of being in good spirits, I suppose. And talk with any of the members? No, one really couldn't or shouldn't bother them. (Maybe a little fear of appearing weak showing up?)

You will probably lose sleep because you wonder what you could do, what you could say, how you could reach them, how you could help, and how to find that magic formula that makes the group members respond. Didn't you present it coherently enough, talking up or down to them?

At other times you will wonder what you did or didn't do, what you had done wrong, why they didn't participate as you had expected them to. Was it your fault? Was your presentation wrong?

And you are probably human enough that you would appreciate a little appreciation for what you do and did—and it's not forthcoming.

Yes, your selfless, willing and glad giving can catch up with you, and you can fall into a caring-burnout, having to look for sources to replenish your strength resources.

It appears to me that maybe term limits would be a good idea? You know, officers would sit out at least a year? But what if nobody is willing to step forward to take over? Will the group fall into disarray and die? Even with the famous 20/20 hindsight, I don't know what the best solution would be.

But basically, yes, support group participation is a rewarding labor of love.

MSWGMD

Getting to newsletter details now. You recall I said I began it with a few personal words. Following are a few examples. The first one is the introduction to newsletter #4:

> How is winter treating you? I hope you like the cold and all the baddies that go along with it. Personally, I hate it! I have declared that white stuff that falls out of the clouds a four-letter word that is not to be uttered in my presence. But I also hate heat and humidity. Poor weather just can't please me.
>
> (But now the beginning of winter 2003/2004 is still six days away; the unmentionable, it is covering the ground three or four inches high, and I hate it!!)
>
> But what I really wanted to talk to you about was something personal. I have trouble talking about myself, talking about my feelings that is, and have chewed on this one for weeks. It still doesn't sound right to me, but I'll

put it before you anyway and hope you'll understand what I'm trying to say.

In April of 1988, I was asked to edit the newsletter for you—although it is more writing than editing it. With some trepidations, I agreed and came to the next meeting.

Well, during my first attendance, I didn't dare getting up, walking around, not even getting me a cup of coffee, although my mouth and throat were straw-dry. I was afraid somebody might laugh at me or pity me. Neither did I dare speaking up because MS has affected my speech and quick thinking. That is, I use a lot of "uh, ah and oh" because finding the right word takes four, five seconds, and at times, it eludes me completely, and I have to talk around it to explain what I'm trying to bring across. Having that left-over German accent doesn't help any. Rather I should say it doesn't help my insecurity any. Anyway, to me, my talking sounds awful, and when I sit a spell too long, my walking gets awful because I've become stiff.

That was my situation in mid -'88. But then I noticed the MSers in wheelchairs—and they didn't look embarrassed. I saw the ones who used canes, crutches and walkers— and they moved around the room freely. I heard people whose speech was affected—and they talked. All in all, neither of these MS persons appeared to be timid, uncomfortable or apologetic; they all acted natural and had fun.

Well, at the May meeting, I had the courage to walk around and dared talking with the lady who sat next to me (she being the one who later became our treasurer and my personal friend). Our chairman asked the question of how we cope. I was the second one to answer and—great surprise to me—without holding back, I could voice my response. After that, I formally joined, for the first time in my life, a group and got actively involved.

I thanked the group members for having helped me along, helped me grow and proceeded on to the write-up of the last meeting.

MSWGMD

After another big ado about an immediate MS cure, I described what I had heard about that latest bovine scatology (borrowed from General Schwartzkopf of Desert Storm fame) and added the following:

News reporters sure are one sensationalistic—uh—bunch aren't they. Everything for a headline that might prick somebody's interest to listen to them or buy the paper or magazine to read the story.

Too bad they don't have to experience on their own bodies and, in their own minds, what they put people through with their awakening false hopes, which, as they know or should know if they were thinking, will be quickly dashed.

And there's not much we can do about that. Or is there? Anyone who has a suggestion, won't you clue me in?"

MSWGMD

The following was the introduction to newsletter # 8:

A couple of days ago, I listened to the weather report, and the meteorologist talked about those dog days. I didn't appreciate the inference that dogs had any connection with these triple H days we're having—hazy, hot and humid. Dogs surely don't deserve that insult.

Yikes, I have to shake my head. Somebody from my family reading this would roar. Nobody who knew me twenty-plus years ago would believe that came out of my pen. All my married life long I had hamsters, till Maxi, our Scottish terrier, that black furball with the expressive brown eyes, wormed himself into my heart in 1974. I was deadly afraid of dogs, but Maxi and his successors changed my mind.

I have often used, and still use, these comforters—dogs, cat, hamsters—as my crying towels when I feel, well, you know, when my body and my life don't treat me as I would like to be treated. The little critters all look so attentive as if they'd understand every word and feel a world full of compassion, which relieves some of the stress and leaves me comforted. And neither of them did or will ever tattle on me.

After Maxi died in '87, my son left his dog Teddy at our house "just till we're settled in in our own home" because the apartment he and his wife rented didn't allow pets. Of course Teddy stayed with us till he died in '94, and after Karlemann, the last hamster, died, I didn't replace him with another one. In '95, our daughter persuaded my husband and me to adopt one of her cat's kittens, and independent Smoky joined our family. Then a neighbor had trouble with her two dogs fighting, so we took Goldie (she's being called the Taco Bell dog) off her hands. At the 2001 Mother's Day, my daughter surprised me with a beautiful midnight blue Siamese fighting fish, but my Sapphire is no fighter; he is a talker and so happy when I turn my chair around and talk with him. Yes, he stands in my office, right next to my desk. (Well, he left me on Easter 2004.)

I hope you, too, have the pleasure of a pet's company.

MSWGMD

During one meeting, we had planned to talk about depression but got sidetracked and just talked the two hours away unstructured, and as usual, that was another quite helpful and productive meeting. That other subject? Well, we could always reschedule it; it, like many other MS symptoms, won't go away nor leave us alone.

That set me to thinking, and in the next newsletter, I wrote the following:

> Multiple sclerosis sure changes one's life so drastically, not only in the negative but also in the positive sense. We adapt to life and the realities of it, I suppose.
>
> Just look at us three officers. Our chairperson had to completely rearrange her life, from being a professional to becoming a handicapped homemaker. She wrote the piece *Forces of the Unknown (Multiple Sclerosis)*. She had to slow down and start to appreciate the world she lived in. Eventually she became our chairperson—and a darn good one, she was.
>
> Our treasurer had it very difficult healthwise. Not only did she have MS, but also diabetes, arthritis, asthma and several other illnesses, each one by itself enough to carry for one person. But she didn't give up. Instead she helped people in her circle of acquaintances and the group members as much as she could with her caring, sympathy and understanding. And her laughter.
>
> After I joined the group, it made me more people-aware. I acted more outgoing and had fun, but mainly, I suppose, it encouraged me to learn more. It made me look into some fascinating subjects, the workings of the brain, the equally wondrous world of the genes, the intricacies of the immune system. In other words, one subject led to another, and the challenge of all that knowledge almost—sorry, only almost—makes up for the inability to take long-stridden walks, to think fast and move fast and having had to give up playing badminton.

MSWGMD

For newsletter #9, I had permission to use a poem about doing good for others, caring for others, helping each other.

I printed that poem first and followed it up with talking along the lines that helping others comes easy for me, but accepting help is the tougher one. But by now I have grown in that area too. An example of then and now.

Our public library and the League of Women Voters sponsor a yearly used book sale and, *oooeeehhh*, did I always clean the psychology section out. In 1989, I chose too much, couldn't lift the box but scooted it along with my good foot. Without asking, several people helped me move that box; two nudged me to go ahead of them in the long line at the cash register.

Was I grateful? Yes, very much so. Did I appreciate the help? Ditto, yes, very much. Did it make me feel good? You want to know the truth? Sorry, no. I felt uncomfortable, embarrassed, even a little ashamed.

I have grown in these dozen years.

Nowadays I can unrestrictedly accept the offered help, as for instance, today at the grocery store I kept dropping things and a young man picked it up. Or somebody holds the door open for me. You know, just extending a little kindness. I can now smile an open, not a grimaced smile, and say: "Thank you; I appreciate it." Some able-bodied people have admitted to me that it makes them feel good when they can help.

MSWGMD

Another "Hi, Everybody" began the New Year.

Well, Christmas is over, 1990 has started, I have finally learned to write the right year on my checks, we had our Christmas-in-January party, and it was another smashing success. In a couple of weeks, we will move into our new home (the group's new meeting place), in a couple of months baseball season will start, and then planting, weeding and vegetable-growth-watching will begin. Yikes, isn't life exciting?

It ain't, huh. At least not always.

Uh, I know what you're talking about. Sometimes it's lousy, depressing, full of anxieties and pessimism. Frequently our good cheer is a pretend job, and sometimes even pretending long enough doesn't convince our mind that we're feeling okay.

But despite all the negativities dished out to us, let's not give up on life just yet. Let's not give multiple sclerosis the upper hand nor let it slow us down permanently, and don't hand it the satisfaction of having defeated us. I have found out that a little prayer does wonders. I mean, something like the following:

A curse...

Well, you darn body (I say rotten, even damn or worse, depending on how bad I feel), I'm tired of this MS causing me this unsteadiness, slowing of mind and body, loss of bladder or bowel control, trembling (insert what gives you the most trouble). I command you to work! I won't let you become the master of my life and over me. It's not you who is in control—I am. and by bleepetybleep, I'm taking the responsibility to stay in charge. You think you can get me down? Ha, you have another think coming. I'm bleepetybleep tired of you giving me all this bleepetybleepbleep trouble. You bleepetybleepbleepbleep understand that?

...And a prayer...

Dear God:

For reasons only known to You, You have let my body be afflicted with multiple sclerosis. I don't like it, but I'll try to accept what You have sent me. Your will be done because I believe You know best what's best for me and I know You won't hand me more than I can handle.

I would greatly appreciate if You would grant me permanent remission, but if that is not in Your plan, at least, I do pray that You give me the courage and strength and the blessings and grace I need to cope with this burden and not collapse under it, especially when I'm depressed and ready to give up.

But please, don't let it become too severe.

Amen.

MSWGMD

Introduction to newsletter #15:

Our Chapter Services Director gave me the idea for this beginning. She talked and showed samples of her hobby—flower arranging—and believe me, they're beautiful works of art. I was thinking that everybody ought to take time out to do something they really like to do, even if it's not perfect, even if it doesn't make any money, but is something done purely for the joy of it, something one can be proud of.

Most of us can wrest a little personal sanctuary out of our house or apartment, a place that is off-limits to the rest of the family, especially the kids. In one of my sixteen so-called permanent addresses as an army wife, I once choose a window at the end of the hallway. In another apartment, I used the corner of the livingroom. In 1975, we bought our house, and I first used the pantry off the kitchen as my office, even if that meant I had to trudge down the stairs in the basement to do the laundry as well as storing and retrieving my canned goods. I had plastered the white-caulked walls around my desk with pretty pictures and greeting cards. The room was so small I could touch the walls around the desk without extending my arms fully, it had just room for my little desk, a chair, the junk shelf and a tea cart with my organ. But it was mine, and I could find pen, paper and notes where I had left them (most of the time anyway).

Then in '92, for our thirtieth wedding anniversary, my husband enclosed the back porch, made two rooms out of it and built me a nice, spacious office with enough room for my large desk, printer table, a couch, the stereo table, two book cases, two hanging cabinets and more. He even had a little space heater installed in the second room, which allows me to use my office even in below-zero temperatures of the Ohio winters. I tell you, it is beautiful, I love it and appreciate it and him.

(After my husband died, the kids were afraid for my safety and nagged me into letting them replace the couch with a bed, and that is where I sleep now most of the time.)

While I'm at it, I'll tell you another story about our Chapter Services Director. In the first few newsletters, I had always talked about MS patients. While readying my little brochure for the printer, she mentioned that we don't act like patients and shouldn't call ourselves that. Then I disagreed with her, grumbled and stubbornly kept on using MS patients.

Over time, I noticed other writers speaking to and about MSers or MS persons and engaged in one of my favorite activities—thinking. My mind kept kicking the idea between the right and the left hemispheres of my brain for a while, and guess what—once again I had to admit that she had been right, darn her. Or was it darn me? Did I think as patients we would beg, steal or borrow more coddling pity parties? Anyway, facts of the matter are that we MSers are too strong, too alive, too proud, have too much fighting spirit and activate too many of our survivor instincts to call ourselves patients.

Darn right I'm proud of us because we're the kinds of persons we are. And since that time, I've been using MSers and MS persons.

MSWGMD

One of our group members mentioned that she had noticed that people didn't act as they had before she came down with MS and wondered whether MS had something to do with it. A few of our members said no to that and asserted it was the world we're living in, that people simply were too self-involved and detached and didn't know any longer how to be friends. (This question has once again come up at one of the MS bulletin boards recently.)

I didn't agree with that when I heard it, and I believe there is more to it than that. I believe we, who have that disease nobody knows much about, do make others uncomfortable. We remind them of illness, suffering and imperfections of body, which, they conclude, also points to an imperfection of mind or soul. That brings on fear, and they retreat into the safety of avoiding us. Facing us might bring on the possibility of them having to face themselves and see life's imperfections. That's too risky.

After all, if it can happen to us, who look so normal, it could happen to them, too, couldn't it? Thus, I say, by avoiding us, they act in support of the principle of "out of sight out of mind" and feel safer.

Also, as I will outline shortly, as much as youth and beauty/handsomeness, fitness, aggressiveness and competitiveness are glorified in our society, we are the odd ones who are not perfect examples of the American ideal.

A third reason: Maybe people are uncomfortable in our presence because they don't know what to say and how to behave. Should they tiptoe around, whisper soothing words as if they were in a hospital room with a dying patient or talk loud in false merriment or be pitying or overly solicitous?

Well, that one we can take care of; make them comfortable by being matter-of-fact. If they want to hear about it, we say a few sentences about having MS and what it does to us, but also stressing what it does not do to us, namely making us invalids who are on the brink of death. It's just that our body doesn't work as it used to and as it is supposed to. Otherwise we act like the persons we are, ask how and what the conversation partner is doing or what they are interested in, you know, engaging in normal-people talk.

Simply solved, isn't it?

MSWGMD

Not all introductions have to be serious, though, nor need they carry a message. Here is the intro to newsletter #23:

Hi, Everybody:

How are you? Better'n I, I hope. No, it's not the MS; I'm pooped from fixing Easter dinner for nine—Cornish game hens, two types of dressing, two vegetables, mashed potatoes (from flakes this time, not from scratch), gizzard gravy, sweet potatoes and a cranberry mold. Not to forget the worst; it was the hottest day to date in this year, and the kitchen was H-O-T, hot. It didn't help that I forgot to open the window till after I was done with the cooking.

But even that didn't floor me—rather chair me. It was what I done did with all that food!!!

U'huh, I'm as stuffed as the hens were and won't have room for dessert till at least eight tonight—if then. Although, thinking about the Peeps and jelly beans and chocolate eggs and, hm…Anyway, I don't want to brag, but sometimes I wish I weren't as good a cook as I am so people wouldn't always hint at wanting to be invited to a meal. Naw, that's not true. As my mother-in-law always said, "The biggest compliment for a cook is when people at her table are eating and seem to enjoy what's on their plate."

And to think, when I got married, I was excellent at opening and heating up a can of convenience food on my two-burner hot-plate, which I had to hide carefully from my landlady. Sometimes I went it fancy and dropped a boil-in-bag-something into boiling water and watched it bubble for the required minutes. Thank goodness my husband's friends gave us an electric percolator as a wedding present, or I'm sure I would've burned the coffee water. Oh, another lady gave me a wonderfully simple and easy-to-follow cook book, which I still use even if it's loose-leafed, brown-paged and food-spattered by now.

Anyway, right now I need an excuse to stay put, and drafting the newsletter is as good a one as any.

I proceeded to the body of the newsletter and ended with:

Well, thanks for listening and helping me take my mind off of me through showing that I was busy. That way my family and guests got their own coffee and dessert, which meant they used the old mugs and everyday dishes instead of the good china, which means it's easier to set them away after I get around to washing 'em.

Oh, by the way, till I met my mother-in-law, I towel-dried my dishes. Well, Mom had no problem persuading me to let them air-dry because, she asserted with a wink, that was more sanitary. Not many people in our family, especially not my husband, object or challenge me when I cite Mom.

You, gentle readers of the younger generation, yes, I admit, that is manipulative, but I'll bet you too will discover a few life-easing shortcuts of your own before you reach the over-fifty bracket.

Okay, that's enough of those entries. I'll now proceed to some...

Tips and Hints

Some people, like me, are afflicted with memory dysfunction. (Doesn't that sound better than plain forgetfulness?) That is, we forget things because thoughts aren't held in our sievy short-term memory long enough to remember from 1/1000th of a second to the next, and the impressions or stimuli aren't forwarded to the long-term memory. In turn we, uh, what did I want to say, ah, I mean, oh yes, I wanted to add that we tend to forget some things.

Through frustrations over forgetting that oh so beautiful or admirable thought, I have trained myself to stop right now and write down any idea worth saving before it disappears into oblivion forever. That's why I have distributed pens and paper in all strategic places in my house (yes, the bathroom too). I have also bought myself a penlight and don't have to turn the lamp on in the night when I want to write something down.

Oh, carrying a micro-cassette recorder around is equally helpful.

But like our CR, I forget that I wrote myself that note or, more likely, forget where I put what I wrote down. She came up with a super-splendiferous idea of throwing a pillow on the floor. When she walks by it, she wonders why the pillow lies there, picks it up and remembers the note.

Well, we are a family of readers; we had books lying around everywhere. (Yes, in the bathroom too; that's why we used to call it the library.) So I used to throw a paperback or a half sheet of scratch paper near where I had dropped a note off. A couple of times during the day, especially in the evening, I pick up books and notes and place the notes in a safe place.

The trouble, though, is that I—did you guess it—forget where that safe place was. I mean, I have two endtables next to my chair in the livingroom, a footstool with cavernous lid-closed storage space, three desks and assorted other drop-off points throughout the house. In turn, I frequently have to run through the house—not literally—like a chicken with its head cut off, wondering where I've left that glorious paper where I'd written down that bleepetybleepbleep result of my brainwork, to, well, just place it in another safe place. (You remember our treasurer's joke about the "hereafter"? Well, that pertains to me quite often—what am I here after?)

Finally I wised up. My sister-in-law is an artist at making canvas items. I asked her to make me a couple of covers (something like book covers) with pockets inside and trained myself to drop the paper slips in there. Sure saves me steps and aggravation.

Talking some more about finding things: I got in the habit of putting everything I frequently use, such as tools, gardening equipment, personal hygiene items, all kitchen thingamajigs—silverware, bowls, plates, utensils, just about everything—in the same place. That way I can find a lot of things much quicker, except when somebody doesn't practice what I not only preach.

While my kids were still at home, and later the grandkids lived at home, I had a heck of a time finding my pens where I needed them till I had a lightbulb go off in my head: I started tying the pens down, one by the phones, one by the bulletin board, one each on the lamp switches and so on.

Ninety percent of them stayed put.

I also have the unsteadiness problem, and bending down to pick something up throws me off balance. Well, I've bought myself some extra-long tongs and pick things up with them.

Two ideas from our CR:

"There are some *super* kitchen tools in some department stores: Extra-wide-handled gadgets with non-slip grips. A little more expensive, but if you watch for sales, not too unreasonable."

She also came up with some nifty ways to use her pizza cutter: "Cut cakes, brownies, pan cookies, even use it to cut homemade noodles."

MSWGMD

My husband had bought a dress shirt, and I'd like to find blouses like that. It has a hidden zipper to close it, and the tiny buttons are only for show, and they needn't be replaced because they are not used.

Wouldn't that be ideal for those of us with clumsy or non-existing fingertips? The manufacturer is "Nifton Super Shirts."

Oh, my daughter-in-law gave me a housecoat with tiny buttons on the outside and hidden big snap closures, which are easier to operate. Thank goodness for thoughtful people.

Yes, putting tiny buttons of blouses or dresses through tiny holes is a tough job. Here is how I do it: I put my thumbnail through the buttonhole, place the button on the inside of it and pull it through. Yes, I still fumble, but experience has helped me to get more efficient at it, and I don't have to ask other people to button things for me.

I have also stopped unbuttoning blouses or tops any longer; I just undo the top one or two buttons and slip it over the head. That eases things too. (Those of you who wear dresses—I'm sure it works for them too. I have given up dresses years ago after discovering slacks to hide my legs in or under. You see, I'm okay with my body generally, but dang it, I don't like my legs, find them too fat, so I found clothes to cover them a blessing.)

One of our group members gave us a tip I still use faithfully and like to pass on. Use plain ole children's Play-Doh to limber up stiff fingers and hands. I had to steal mine from my grandson while he was younger, and he kept wondering what was in that brown jar he wasn't allowed to open. U'huh, he might have stolen it back or steal it now for his little brother.

For Women Only: A fairly newly diagnosed lady asked how we hooked our bras. One lady said she had replaced all her back-snapping ones with front-closures, but many do what I do: Turn it around, fumble the hooks shut, pull it around and slip my arms through the straps. It requires a little body wiggling but beats getting stiff arms from blindly groping to match hooks and eyelets in the back.

MSWGMD

Okay, I want to end this segment with a talk about something that is extremely helpful but also can be extremely difficult for some of us.

I bet you agree that gadgets, electric utensils and power tools are easing our lives, make the work go faster and more efficient. And when we have a headache, be it a splitting one or one just waiting in the wings to attack us, we take a pain reliever, now don't we, huh, huh, don't we?

If you answered with a pitying, impatient or condescending "Of course," implying that I asked a stupid question, I follow that up with the next question to those who refuse to use mobility aids: Why don't you wear that brace, use a cane, walker, crutches or wheelchair?

Let's start with the braces. There are quite a few different ones around. Some are made of sturdy plastic, starting from under the balls of the foot, supporting the ankle and the whole backside of the leg ending just below the kneecap. Others cover sole of foot to the ankle, have two straps on both sides of the leg and fasten with velcro under the kneecap. Yet others, the newer ones, are sort of foam or air-filled. No matter the type, they are designed to keep the ankle and/or knee stable, prevent their buckling under and causing painful falls. The part under the sole of the foot keeps the toes from curling under and causing a fall, something many MS persons, myself included, are prone to do.

Yep, some of them look ungainly, and I know some MSers hate to wear them with shorts or dresses, but dang it, if they help, let's just wear slacks or pantsuits. That's what I do, even when I go with my son to his church, and I don't feel bad when I'm the only woman who has her legs covered. I'm usually also the only one who uses a cane or a walker.

Mobility aids have many plus-points going for them. People who use them fall down less, and it's safer for walls and furniture because one bumps into them less often. Those thingies keep the user more independent, and it's nothing to be ashamed of; it's shameful only if one sees it as such. Also, one gets less pooped out, can go to more places and expends less energy going from point A to point B.

It took some time until I had worked myself through to this acceptance ,but age, self-acceptance and MS-acceptance have made me wiser and more sensible, to the point that now I can speak in the third person; that is, excluding myself from this advice because I took it. The advice, I mean. As I have mentioned earlier, I do use the cane, while in exacerbations I used the walker, and for longer outings, I do climb, without too many qualms, in the wheelchair—the manual ones that I can operate myself, which gives that sense of being in control.

No, it was not easy to overcome my pride of what I considered advertising that I'm handicapped, but when I started torkeling around as if I were drunk, I used a regular cane to stabilize myself. Next I advanced to the quad cane for added stability. I still use it when I leave the house.

I do carry the cane in my right hand and noticed that I had more and more trouble with the right side of my body and suspected that it stemmed from leaning on the cane. My chiropractor confirmed that that might be quite likely. During the next visit with my neurologist, he advised me strongly to proceed to a walker. I acceded.

I did like the security and ease of the walker, but it had one drawback. Between seven in the morning (when I get up) till midnight (when I go to bed), I make some dozen or more trips to the kitchen and hated like heck to have somebody wait on me, bringing me my coffee or food.

Well, I solved my problem by getting a small thermos and attached a plastic shopping bag on my walker. I filled the thermos, put it in the bag and filled my coffee cup after I had sat down again. Worked like the oft-cited charm. As my daughter-in-law said: "The best inventors are those who need it." A little later, my sister-in-law gave me a walker with a basket, which I can attach or remove when I go somewhere.

A little warning is in order. Yes, it is easier and more convenient to climb in the wheelchair or scooter—even if it's not truly needed. Please don't get me wrong, but I do know people who are feeling sorry for themselves and baby their MS. Some do use the illness as a crutch to avoid doing things or doing things for themselves. Through mustering their strength and using that little extra effort, some of them could get out of the wheelchair and be more independent. But most MS people I know won't let the disease get them down; they stay as mobile, independent and self-sufficient as they possibly can.

If eventually I do need the wheelchair, though, permanently or because the darn immune system has done too much permanent damage, I know I will be able to accept it. Four people in our group had done so, and I admired how factually they accepted their condition.

So why not reconsidering? As soon as you get better, you can blow the cane/walker/wheelchair a kiss or stick your tongue out at it and ban it to the corner closet, the attic or the basement.

MSWGMD

There is no good place to put the following, so I will just put it here.

Sad to say, many good things in life come to an end—and so did my association with the group. Eventually the group itself ended.

I had some major disagreement with the Chapter; they wanted more control over the running of the group, but the treasurer and I wanted to keep independent as we had been for all these successful years. Two factions within the group pulled in the different directions—dependence on the Chapter versus independence. Power struggles were going on big time, envy and jealousy raised their ugly heads, and lies were being told. So in the summer of 1993, to retain my self-respect, sanity and escape from the conflicts tearing at my mind and soul, I decided to resign. Two months later, our treasurer resigned too; she couldn't take any longer what they had made of the group. I attended one meeting but was not made welcome by the new leadership and stopped going, just kept in contact with a few of my friends.

In May 1994, I received the following form letter: "The Crawford County Multiple Sclerosis Support Group will no longer hold meetings. This is due to a lack of interest and poor attendance…"

It is now over ten years since I received this letter. Our CR and I are still in contact. (Sadly though, this is restricted to exchanging Christmas greetings. She is not feeling well healthwise, and I'm so darn busy.) Three ladies attend the same church I attend, and we talk occasionally. Our treasurer and I stayed friends until she passed on. Two other ladies and I exchange e-mails. I still end my correspondence to MSers or my postings on the bulletin boards as I always did: "Best wishes for permanent remission."

But yes, I'm still sad and still miss our group.

MSWGMD

I'd like to end this chapter with a few personal words and hope you won't accuse me of being preachy, mean-spirited or high-horse-ish. I'll just tell you how I try to live my life.

Yes, I'm somewhat hindered in accomplishing all the necessary tasks and need others to help me out occasionally. I have learned to accept that help graciously, without feeling humiliated, ashamed or taking advantage of others. It took some time, but now I'm confident enough about myself to even ask for needed help.

On the other hand, I won't let others do too much for me, don't let them take over my life, my responsibilities or let them do what I very well can do for myself and by myself. That is, I won't get lazy and ask others to do what I, with a little extra effort, can do myself. I just take care not to overdo nor to underdo. (Of course I do slip up occasionally. Don't we all?)

A German proverb exhorts a person to "*Nicht Kapital draus schlagen.*" In regards to MS, it can be used to mean "not using the illness for illicit gains."

I try not to dwell on what I can't do, but perfect, refine and strengthen what I can do, not focusing on my limits but on my strengths, not being a giver-upper but a fighter. Mind you, I say limits not limitations.

And let's not worry too much about the future. I'm sure you have heard about the self-fulfilling prophecies. With over-worrying, we might bring on what we fear. I try to live each day as best as I can and take care of the future when it turns into the present.

And I definitively do not feel sorry for myself any longer. At least not for long. I get angry, yes, and frustrated and irritated, but I will not let self-pity take over and hamper me from getting the best out of life.

I do wish that being a fighter won't be made too difficult for you, that MS won't bring you to your knees—except to pray—nor set you on your rear. Just never, never ever, give up or give up hope.

I know that's easy to say, but God Almighty, is it tough to live it. Keeping the will to live is easy; keeping on to function, to fight, fight depression, rebuff the temptation to lay down and play dead—that is the tough part.

I know. I have been there and will get there again. I had eye trouble, feared it might be MS-related, but thank God, it was only my cataracts acting up, something that could be remedied with surgery. During the pre-op times and while recuperating, I was unable to read, write or work on the computer, which put me in the dumps for a while.

But basically I keep trying and hope you will too. Keep trying, I mean. Even if sometimes it's a one step forward and three back affair. Just let's not give up on ourselves and our lives. I repeat it all the time: I will not give multiple sclerosis the satisfaction of having defeated me.

MSWGMD

That ends the theoretical part. In the next chapter I would like to talk about living at peace with ourselves, with others and with multiple sclerosis.

Chapter Six
Living, Coping, Accepting and a Little Psychology

In the last chapter I mentioned the health versus illness issue and would like to expand on what I said there.

Our fast-paced society over-glamorizes people who are young, energetic, risk-taking go-getters. Middle and older age is abhorred. So-called oldsters arouse pity, impatience and rejection. I read on 14 May 2002 that even medical students hold to that opinion—and that is putting it mildly; the paper used much stronger words, something like thinking poorly about older Americans.

Those who are physically disabled are classified as not-perfect. I repeat what I said before—I strongly believe this recoiling from the ill and infirm is fear-based. Facing the aged and ill ones makes people uneasy because it brings into awareness their own vulnerability. They realize they, too, are vulnerable, could fall victim to illness, lose zest, vim and vigor. Men see being ill as losing machismo, especially those with names like Joe Macho Doe or Don Grabber Upclawer. Women with names like Jill Beauty Queen or Wanda Want It All find it difficult to cope with a physical impairment. And we won't forget those men or women who are named Chris Damaged Merchandise or Tony Giverupper.

As I see it, aging and illness frightens, in particular, those who let society and its current trends determine their self-image, their outlook on life and the people in it. They act, react and interact in manners they believe conform to standards which have been declared to be the norms of normal. When people can't live up to what they think the world expects they ought, should or must do to be acceptable, or when they get attacked with something like multiple sclerosis, they flee those who are no longer good enough.

At the bottom line of this behavior lies the fear that interacting with the handicapped or the aged could bring the same dreadfulness about even quicker.

Ergo and in short, being ill-physically, intellectually or emotionally, just doesn't fit the picture of what the normal American should be like or should do. Thus those who consider themselves to be the healthy ones turn away from those who, well, you fill in the blank please.

What makes it even worse, though, is the fact that not only healthy people put the ill ones down, some of those not in perfect health believe they no longer fit the norm and do tremendous hatchet jobs on themselves. They lose their self-worth feelings to the point that they need sump pumps to get them out of the basement of wretchedness. This self-vilification brings on additional spiritual or emotional components like despair, depression, giving up and loneliness.

Yes, we do get hurt, intimidated, shrink back, doubt ourselves to the point that we miss out on life and what it still has to offer us because we let others determine our worth and value as persons.

But not for long. We strong ones we will not let that get us down. You see, we can't give up in discouragement, dispiritedness and despair because there is so much to do and only we, you and I, can do it. For instance, there are:

- prayers to pray.
- original thoughts to think and convey to others.
- new things to learn and discover and stimulate others to build on them.

- articles, books and poems to read and write.
- works of art to paint.
- beauties to see.
- young and old to teach.
- music to listen to and to compose.
- imperfections to correct.
- money to spend.
- birds, chipmunks, butterflies and fishes to watch and be amused by.
- nature to admire.
- battles to win.
- uglies to change.
- good deeds to do.
- challenges to meet and overcome.
- goodness to praise.
- people to thank and praise.
- resolutions of not giving up to keep.
- discussions to hold, standpoints to defend.
- comfort to dispense.
- listening with the ears of the soul.
- minds to sharpen.

And a million other things are waiting to be done, to see, to smell, to speak, to sense and to hear. And a lot of it is waiting for you to accomplish.

See? You can't give up. There is too much to do.

MSWGMD

Now let me offer for your perusal some insights which are designed to stimulate self-awareness and Self-awareness. I believe, whether we are healthy or ill, we all can benefit from a program of self-discovery, which also aids greatly in understanding others and makes living with ourselves and them a tat easier.

P.S. to that paragraph: My triple D (dear darling daughter) objected to the word "perusal" and insisted I include a definition of it. Following that order, I will say that perusal means thinking something through, considering it, working on it mentally. But you knew that already, didn't you?

At first I had planned to use the "A" Ladder in a spirituality project (in the note-taking stage), but I will offer an abbreviated version to you first. The other three pieces I wrote originally as an aid in my novel writing, to better understand the characters I had created, but eventually I expanded that to better understand myself and others and make it a tat easier to respectfully live with them and myself.

Here is an introduction in the phraseology I use:

"Self"capitalized: The person we really are, inside and out.
Wantneeds: Things we'd like to have but can survive without.
Inner and Outer Life: The life we appear to live, the life others see versus the life of our thought world, the two often being opposites.
Public and Private Face: The Self we show to others, the Self we really are, the Self we think we are.
Motivators: That's shorthand for our hidden goals. They influence how we act, react and interact with ourselves and others, how we want to be treated or seen by others—being liked and admired, be rich, powerful and in control, being taken care of and so on.

Here is the "A" Ladder :

The "A" Ladder
Aims
Amusement
Approval
Allowance
Abundance
Admiration
Association
Appeasement
Activities
Affection
Adequateness
Appreciation

This "A" Ladder depicts what I believe people would like to receive from others and from their feelings about themselves. These wishes can turn to expectations, up to becoming must-haves. No matter how weak or how strong these motivators are, they influence our reactions to life, situations we encounter, responses to what confronts us in our life; simply said, what influences our actions, reactions and interactions.

For instance, consider Abundance-seekers. One is a little greedy; the other a little miserly; a third spends money a little too impulsively; a fourth values personal possessions; a fifth is stingy with her/his time; the sixth hates to share thoughts. That makes none of them a despicable person, just somebody who is human and has a few little human quirks. As I said, it depends on the degree and is all right as long as it does not get wide-ranging. There are quite a few different motivators available to choose one's behavior style from with the major goal of the exercise leading to the result of Self-awareness.

Each person on God's sometimes-not-so-pretty earth is an individual, and as such, each of us has their personal goals of what we wish to receive in our life; we pursue these goals in our own personalized way, going so far as to push toward excesses in either direction.

A few explanatory words for each motivator:

Abundance—having things.
Activities—having something to do, searching for variety.
Adequateness—wanting to be at least as good as others, preferably being better, searching for self-esteem and a feeling of self-worth.
Admiration—having or doing something to be proud of, having that acknowledged by others through praise.
Affection—being liked and loved, being able to love oneself, having someone to be close to, belonging to somebody.
Aims—having goals, aspirations, dreams, caring for something, seeking success.
Allowances—giving in, not thinking too highly of oneself.
Amusement—wanting to have fun, not having to expend too much energy or effort on the dreariness of life, avoiding thinking.

Appeasement—wanting to live at peace with oneself and others, avoiding fights, having few worries and low anxiety levels.

Appreciation—receiving gratitude, having one's good deeds duly acknowledged.

Approval—being respected, well, simply being approved of by oneself and others.

Association—having friends and acquaintances, not being alone and lonely.

The "A" Ladder in Detail

People, being different from each other, are motivated by different goals. These motivators color actions, reactions and interactions and make us behave as we do.

For instance, some people value their privacy, want to live at peace in quiet surroundings. Their motivator is appeasement. Others seek action, excitement, adventure in life's fast lane. Their motivators are Activities and Amusement.

I believe most people to a greater or lesser degree search for the fulfillment of the life qualities this "A" Ladder depicts and would like to reap the benefits associated with them. The manner in which they are going for their goals illustrates what is commonly called what makes us tick, which means individual people give their main motivators highest priority.

I do not imply that these motivators typify people, that all people with a common motivator pursue exact same goals. As I have said, all of us being individuals, we may have the same motivator—say Admiration—but we all differ in the application of pursuing our objectives.

I would like to invite you to look these motivators over, think about them and honestly, without over-valuing nor under-valuing yourself, judge if and to what degree you express the behavior patterns described.

If you decide to discuss these evaluations with another person and they express some conclusion about you and your personality, reserve for yourself the final judgment as regards truth or falsehood of the appraisal. You know yourself, and with a little practice, you can become honest with yourself, minimizing the little discomforts when self-praise is due.

Of course this list reflects my thinking while you want to add, subtract or discard what does not fit your style or what does not pertain to you. That is perfectly all right.

A tip: Most of us are in the habit of judging ourselves too harshly, seeing our minus points and overlooking the plus points. Maybe your analysis sounds too negative, too gloomy, with the emphasis being on not-so-wholesome aspects of the personality traits which, thus, have to be squirreled away from self- and other-awareness.

Let's revisit, reconsider, reevaluate that. In all my counseling, writing, even cajoling, I advocate the qualities of clarity of thinking (honest self-examination), self-acceptance (accepting ourselves as the person and personality we are with all our good sides and liabilities) and self-love (loving ourselves as the person and personality we are while trying to be the best person we can be).

MSWGMD

What did you think? Who did you find out about?" Did you think: Well, oho, aha and haha, here's Dad, Mom, my spouse, Bro, Sis, clear's a bell." Or: "Hm, so that's what Auntie seeks," or "So that's why Unc acts that-a-way.

Now, uh, how about a focus-turn-around? You know, reversing viewpoints and glancing at the lists once more but this time asking: "Is that how I act, or do I act in the opposite manner?" which is the same nickel, dime or quarter—just the other side of it. It is really helpful to find out everything we can about the most important person in our lives—ourselves—to help us live with ourselves and get along better with others.

Now the other three pieces:

About People
People Are Individuals

People—they look different, act different, like and dislike different things, but they all have wantneeds, an inner and an outer life, a public and a private face.

People—they love and hate, talk and think, play and worry, succeed and fail, face blessings and conflicts, have strengths and weaknesses, hopes and fears, are caring and thoughtless.

People—they want to live at peace with themselves, in harmony with others, while trying to achieve their motivators.

Some people feel valuable only after others have affirmed them as such; they accept themselves only after others show them that they are acceptable; they need to see themselves, as the old cliche goes, reflected in an other's eyes,

As I said so many times, people are different. Some bend over backwards to be liked, to fit in, be approved of. Others care less about what others think about them. Some are subjective, and some are objective. Some like to touch, and others shrink away from human contact. Some are thinkers, and others are doers, and…and…

But all people are individuals in their own rights and have to be respected as such. These individuals can and should claim the right to live their lives as they see fit—as long as that does not infringe on the rights of others.

Life requests of us that we mature, grow, work ourselves through to making up our own minds; within naturally imposed limits we do what we like, refuse to do what we dislike or what interferes with our principles, values and beliefs. And we stand up for these our principles, values and beliefs.

Our relationships with others are important. Being selfish, self-focusing, self-centered, thinking only about oneself, expecting others to give to us and cater to us puts us and them in the emotional poorhouse.

Some people are givers, and some are takers, and both harm themselves through their excesses. To live a balanced life, we have to both give and take, thinking about others but equally thinking about ourselves, do things for others and do things for ourselves.

My Prescription for Living

The following may seem like an exorbitantly long list, it being impossible to ever achieve it all, but don't turn away from it in disgust please; at least look it over. I haven't mastered all the points either. Some I will, personality-wise, be unable to ever achieve. But we can always learn, strive and improve ourselves, at least partially. And I bet you, as well as I, do a lot of that automatically already.

But through thinking (along with reading, learning and writing being my favorite activity) I have learned one thing, and that is accepting responsibility for what I do and don't do, what I can do and can't do. Since learning and living that life lesson, I rarely blame others for what I am responsible for. But neither do I blame myself or accept blame for something I don't need to feel guilty about. I just accept that I am an imperfect human being, living in an imperfect world among other imperfect human beings.

Life can be easier if we learn to live with some of the following principles:

*Being persistent, not giving up.
*Asking questions and asking for help when needed.
*Being optimistic.
*Not abusing oneself or others, whether physically or verbally, even when one hurts.
*Having the courage to admit that one has made a mistake.
*Not being afraid to be honest, vulnerable and interdependent.
*Not thinking one has to be perfect because—besides God—nobody is perfect.
*Having the courage to freely say "yes" or "no."
*Accepting constructive criticism but rejecting abuse.
*Believing in oneself, in one's right to pursue the goals of liberty and happiness in one's personal, individualized way.
*Having confidence in oneself.
*Determining one's own lifestyle.
*Being honest with oneself about oneself and practicing honesty in interactions with others.

*Loving oneself unconditionally, with all one's strengths and weaknesses.
*Looking inside oneself for one's life orientation.
*Being proud of oneself.
*Respecting oneself and others.
*Accepting responsibility for one's actions, reactions and interactions.
*Feeling and believing that one is a worthy individual.

Accepting oneself honestly with all one's strengths and weaknesses is really not that bad, now is it?

If you don't mind, I'll stick with this subject for a bit longer and ask the following question:

How Do You Feel

Mentally, I mean. Are you contented, satisfied, at peace with yourself and the world? Or are you angry, fearful, depressed, worried, feeling sorry for yourself? What would you say if I told you that you feel as you choose to?

That it's b.s. and what else?

The truth. That's what it is. The truth. We are not helplessly at the mercy of our thoughts, feelings and emotions. At least to some extent we can be masters of them and control them. I'm a strong believer in the power of thinking. I think about what happens to me, in my world, in my life. I consider it, evaluate it, ask questions about it and answer my questions as honestly as I can.

No, that doesn't put baby blue and cherry pink clouds over my head; the not-so-pleasant parts of my life are still with me. I still have the health problems of multiple sclerosis and arthritis. Other problems of living, for instance relationship problems, attack me as they attack everybody else. Worries try to get me down, have to be fought with—and that gets rough, tough and tumble, sometimes too often.

But most of the time I'm able to use my fighter's clarity of thinking, responsibility-taking and acceptance, as I call them, to help me deal with what life dishes out to me. Incidentally, that is part of my daily prayer for myself and others.

What I wanted to say, though, is that I appreciate and am highly grateful for this great gift of being able to think and have free will to decide. It is thinking and how we respond to what happens that determines how we feel.

Following is the formula of how I see thinking's role as affecting and determining mood, attitude and feelings.

(Yes, gentlemen, you are addressed too. I speak of legitimate feelings which express our humanness, not what you may derisively snort at as fe-e-e-h-minine fe-e-e-e-h-h-h-hlngs.)

A. Something happens. (A new MS symptom appears, or a familiar one worsens.)

B. You recognize it. (You become aware of it.)

C. You analyze it. (You determine what it means.)

D. You evaluate it. (You determine what it means to you.)

E. You interpret it. (You develop a feeling-response about it—anger, hate, worry, fear, self-pity, resignation, depression.)

F. (a) You respond to it. (You feel sorry for yourself; you worry, are angry, are certain that it's the beginning of the end, curse yourself and your body, give up.)

Or,

F. (b) You respond to it. (Knowing you had several exacerbations followed by remissions, you accept it, not happily or shouting for joy from the rooftops, but accepting it you do, as factual as you can, making the best of the given situation, expect it to get better, adjust your life till the improvement occurs.

By the way, this formula can be used for any life situation encountered.

Of course as soon as you are clear-minded you will realize that option "F. (a)" causes a lot of stress, which can do no good, just make things worse.

Explanation of the Formula

"A" is not under our conscious control. Some things we'd much rather not happen to us, but often we get them handed to us whether we like it or not. But the reaction to it is up to us. We can learn to accept and make the best of a bad situation. With thinking and through thinking, we can do that.

"B," "C" and "D" are important, of course, to analyze the whole picture. "E" is the precursor of "F," and all five are filtered through our personal life experiences, with mood and attitude depending whether we chose "F (a)" or "F (b)."

Here is, simplified, why I say that we feel as we choose to feel. Everything that happens, whether initiated by us or others, each thought we think, each action we take, each incident we experience impresses itself on our conscious awareness and evokes an emotional response—we like it or dislike it; it pleases or disturbs us; we define it as good or bad. This judgment then influences our way of viewing the incident, ourselves, our life and the people in it. It also determines our corresponding reaction and action.

Well, I'm sure you believe, as I do, that not only the immune system doesn't like it if we let something depress us, worry us, dispirit us; our mind rebels too when we make negative "F (a)" choices and sink in the dumps instead of thinking realistically, keeping up the fighting spirit, not giving up and mainly making rational, logical, realistic "F (b)" choices.

To test my theory about the power of observation-feeling, emotion and response connection, just think back.

How did that favorite room in your house or a place in your yard or any scenery on God's pretty earth look to you; how did you communicate with yourself and others while you were satisfied with your life and contented with your circumstances?

How did that same place look after you experienced an exacerbation, had a disagreement with somebody or somebody hurt your feelings? Quite a difference in the way things look, isn't there? Ergo, as I said, we are in charge of how we feel, even if it depends on how life, other people and especially we ourselves treat us.

Living Versus Coping

In the manuscript of my other non-fiction work titled *Coping with Life and the People in It*, the right hemisphere of my brain kicked in and told me *Living with MS* is a misnomer. We live with a spouse, parents and children. We interact with other family members, friends, acquaintances, even strangers.

But multiple sclerosis, we have to cope with and that coping is more than mere living with it. To me, learning to live with MS is passive putting-up-with-it-ness. It's a case of takin' it. Life is in charge of us instead of it being the other way around.

Coping with MS, on the other hand, is active in-charge-ness. It puts us at the controls. It is acting, not reacting, doing, not enduring, and gives the strength to expend that extra effort to do a bit more than we thought we were capable of and doing it without getting exhausted from over-doing.

MSWGMD

In my newsletter #12, the one that said "Happy Easter" on the front page, I sent out a salvo of full-fledged attacks on our members. If the projectiles hit their target and people did the thinking, I don't know. Here is what I wrote:

> With spring being officially here, at least according to the calendar, many people think about spring housecleaning. You might be one of those who enjoys that activity, or be more like me, those who put it off till they can see…Uh, I better not remind myself. [As I wrote that the first time I had just gotten my house ready for meeting my nephew's wife, and let me tell you, that was almost as bad as being murdered. That was then, in 1996; now that she has been here three times, she is part of the family and knows my housecleaning practices and seems comfortable with its disorderly order.]
>
> Anyway, [I continued in the newsletter] no matter which group you belong to, I'd like to invite you to do some mental housecleaning.

"How to get about that?" you ask. I'll gladly tell you, because I'm quite familiar with it, having practiced it and still practicing it frequently over the years.

You begin with (a) deciding which area you want to work on. (You ask yourself questions about yourself, your actions, reactions, interactions and non-action..) You (b) assemble the tools and equipment. (You do a lot of thinking about the questions.)

Then comes the tough part, the scouring and scrubbing. That is, you evaluate what you found in (a) and (b) even if it smarts because you discover that you're not as grand and admirable as you thought you were. You even continue if you discover that you're grander and more admirable than you'd given yourself credit for and fear that you are deceiving yourself. And you keep going if you discover that the answers demand a change in attitude and behavior and even if change ranks for you right alongside or behind grumbling and growling and barking about that blarney MS.

Finally you apply the finishing touches; you accept yourself as you are, with all your strengths and weaknesses, all your successes and failings, all your capabilities and limits.

Here are some sample questions I use to stimulate my mind to come up with answers designed specifically for me.

*Do I value myself as a worthwhile individual?
*Do I do what I think I should do or what I truly want to do?
*Do I believe I'm worthy enough to be loved and do I love myself unconditionally?
*Do I accept myself as the person I am while trying to improve what could stand improvement?
*Am I my own best friend and, as such, treat myself with courtesy, respect and loving-kindness?

*Am I in the bad habit of putting myself down while elevating others?

*Or do I do the opposite by elevating myself and putting others down?

*What is my goal in acting, reacting and interacting with others—do I seek acceptance, approval, admiration or any of the other items from the "A" Ladder?

*Do I save my dignity, integrity and self-respect through working toward self-acceptance, self-approval and self-love?

And the important one:

*Do I realize I am the most important person in my life?

That's right. That's what you are. Just think. If you weren't here, the world, your family, friends and all the people you come in contact with would be poorer for it.

Do you also know who our best friend is, the one who has our very best interest at heart, who is always there for us, is happy to talk with us and listen to us?

It's our true Self. It might be buried under lots garbage (putting ourselves down, thinking poorly about ourselves, seeing mainly our imperfections instead of the many good qualities we possess). Yes, sometimes we have to dig a little deeper to unearth that true Self of ours, but it is there, waiting for us, and it really would be only too happy to be of assistance to us.

MSWGMD

Let's also talk about the people who tell you what you, for your own good, ought, should and must do. Reject that. Reject it soundly. Tell them in, uh, words you are comfortable with and calling up the factual strength necessary to bring your point across, that you can manage well enough on your own. Tell 'em that, yes, you may be physically impaired, but by gosh by gum by golly, your mind is working fine, thank you. And since you are more sedentary, you have even more time to think things through to their logical conclusion.

Of course I realize some of us depend on others—caregivers for instance—and we have to be silent about our thoughts to keep their good will; thus we are unable to voice our honest opinions. But at least we can use our freedom of thought and soothe ourselves with the thought that we accept what we can't change. I always say the AA Prayer is not for alcoholics alone. Every person can benefit from its wisdom.

MSWGMD

I had mentioned another subject I would like to talk about in a little more detail, that big hold-up that prevents action-taking for many people—it being shying away from change.

You say your energy is being used up by mere living? Or you point to the old hat of the canine, which, because of its age, is unable to acquire proficiency in novel skills. (Yes, I used the Thesaurus for this sentence.) In other words, do you assert that you are too set in your ways to successfully attempt and complete a comprehensive life-turn-around? Or is change, in your opinion, just too much of a bother without significant rewards?

Well, let me tell you, I (and I think I mentioned it before) am a stubborn, set-in-my-ways-of-doing-and-thinking Taurus, and according to my family, friends and neighbors, it's tough to change my mind. Yet I consider myself living proof that change, even (maybe especially) after age fifty, is possible and dang rewarding. After I turned fifty, I consciously changed more in, on and around me than in the previous twenty-five years combined.

After psychology snared me in and I increased my knowledge, I changed a lot of my mental outlook and carried that over into physical change after I joined the group. My daughter was nonplused when she observed me there and said, "Mami, I can't believe it; you're a completely different person here."

She was right. I could talk, state my opinions and defend them, walk around, approach and speak with different people, even strangers. Maybe I'm a more outgoing personality than I had believed to be all my life? I don't know. It just happened; I let it happen, encouraged it after I recognized the merits and extended it to the broader sphere of my life. It sure has enriched my life, reduced some resentment-stress and grudge-holding and increased life- and people-acceptance.

Does that sound as if I had turned assertively outspoken, standing up for myself and my rights? Nope, I'm not there yet and will not get there completely. (I almost said never, but I'm afraid I'm still holding back myself, just having changed sufficiently to ease my life a bit.) Especially I changed my thinking about myself.

But after my husband's death I did learn to stand more on my own feet, did my own deciding, did my own calling of authorities. I made a mistake or two, but that's okay; I smoothed it out in the end.

MSWGMD

I'd like to use the rest of this book to relate a few more personal experiences, share some observations, thoughts and ideas and hope they can provide you with help in coping with that thing called multiple sclerosis.

I will begin with three personal experiences:

1. In general, I have and had a fairly endurable course of MS, responding well to Lioresal, Prednisone and Avonex. That is, I can cope with and adapt to the restrictions and limits it imposes on me. In December of 1992, though (ten year anniversary of MS diagnosis, some good and a major amount of bad stress) a major exacerbation hit, a lot of this was plainly visible, and for once, I talked honestly with my family about my problems.

About a week into that exacerbation, I tried to rescue two pies from sliding out of the oven; one of them landed on my hand onto the floor, and, uh, you wouldn't have wanted to hear the undeleted expletives I uttered. In other words, I burned my right hand, it hurt, and I cursed loudly and with gusto, most of it in English. (I think I mentioned that usually, when I have time to think before using profane language, I utter said expletives in German, but at that time, I did it in, let's say, raw English.)

After a couple of days, that burn decreased to being a mere nuisance and didn't prevent me from cooking, doing laundry, dishes and typing. But my family kept inquiring about the status of my hand, while it was the flare-up symptoms that hit the hardest and made me feel, uh, lousy.

It wasn't that they were thoughtless or inconsiderate; I see it as a matter of them not understanding. MS doesn't show; hearing an MSer talk about the disease doesn't evoke an illness image. When people hear that somebody has cancer, diabetes, arthritis, had an operation, has a cut or burn, people have an idea of what goes in or on the body of that patient. With MS, it isn't that clear-cut.

But listen to this: About six days into this, one of our group members happened to call. Instantly I felt less depressed, felt a special kind of kinship and relief. I knew I could talk with him and he would understand what I was talking about.

MSWGMD

Just before Thanksgiving 2001, I was hit with a powwow of a doozie of the Big E. Besides all the familiar symptoms, vertigo added itself to it. I reviewed the past few weeks and noted the stressors that had led up to it.

Yes, stress. Remember, I define it as any too much—be that a good thing or a bad one. Both, in my opinion, are equally stressful.

Equally, in my opinion, I believe stress is at least part of the Factor X trigger—and I don't care if the National, the Chapter and some neurologists disagree with me. I know what happened and happens to me and to several other MS persons I know or talk with on the MS bulletin boards. Quite a few doctors and scientists hold that stress does play a role in aggravating the immune system and bringing on flare-ups.

The moral of this: Staying vigilant has its benefits. We don't need to overly concentrate on what goes on in our life, but staying on guard brings major benefits. When I know I will face a particularly stressful time (as for instance preparing that big bash to honor my daughter's graduation from college or having to approach somebody I know I will have an argument with or being warned by the caller ID of a detestable phone call I'm extra cautious before and after), I take my vitamins and medications more faithfully and sit down for two or three spells instead of one.

And of course I arm myself with courage, don't give in to being too dispirited for longer than, say, an hour or two, turn to my God, asking Him for the help I need. Yes, I strongly believe in the power of prayer, for myself as well as for others.

We discussed that feeling un-understood in group one evening, using it as an example and an exhortation to call on another MSer when we know he or she is feeling not so good. We know, and they know we know, what we are talking about because we all go through the same thing, even if the symptoms differ.

MSWGMD

I opened up another subject for discussion, namely whether to talk with family and friends, how much and what to say. I don't mean talking about nothing but one's suffering nor being so pseudo-heroic as to refuse to talk about the Big It at all. Both attitudes are defective.

Here is what we came up with: Those MS persons with an MS-accepting attitude feel free to talk and do so factually without over- or under-reporting, without being ashamed, embarrassed or uncomfortable. They simply state how they feel in body, mind, soul and spirit.

We also agreed on another item: We who have that illness, which most people don't know much about, can be made to feel like outcasts, ashamed, curiosity-attracting, made to feel worth less than so-called healthy people.

Many illnesses arouse pity; some evoke fear; others cause people to avoid contact with the ill person. MSers somehow get all three of the above—and more. After coming to grips with the facts, though, one reaches the point where this only brings a pitying and amused grin.

Told you our group members were smart ones.

MSWGMD

Now the second personal story, explaining why I'm so fascinated with endorphins. I believe they are not only pain relievers—and the medical community acknowledges now that there is pain involved in MS—I'm convinced they also contribute to a person's general well-being.

After I had familiarized myself with the subject as much as was possible with the limited literature available, I began watching myself, especially after the instance of what I am convinced of were endorphin highs and lows.

We three officers prepared for our first Christmas-in-January party, and I was really excited about it. I felt great for days, not too much MS troubles at all; my left arm and leg worked okay, and even the brain didn't make me search for too many words too often, but functioned nearly normal. Fatigue came less frequent and responded to shorter rest periods.

At the party, we had a great turnout, did a lot of talking, laughing and calorie-laden eating. I could walk straight lines and needed the cane more for guidance than support.

The party ended; my family and I came home; I set the left-over food away, piled the dishes in the sink and sat down in my chair.

All of a sudden, I felt drained, without energy and strength, fatigued with a capital F. And all the other MS tweaks and pings, they hit full force too. All I wanted to do was lay my head back, stretch my legs out and take a nap.

But this time I decided not to give in but do something. What? Read? No, my mind wasn't that receptive. Do the dishes? Heck no, I wasn't that desperate. I just pulled my lap desk over and sketched the next chapter of the project I was working on at the time. And you know something? Since I did something I enjoyed and felt challenged by, I could concentrate and think logically; my mind cleared up, and pretty soon I could work effectively.

Since then, I have availed myself regularly to these self-motivators, and it still works.

Yes, endorphins are an MSer's best friend.

MSWGMD

As my third personal testimony, I want to discuss a subject some of you may not want to hear about, it being death, dying and the afterlife. If you feel uncomfortable reading about that, feel free to go to the next section.

We three officers participated in a health fair and met the executive director of the Tri-County Hospital, a wonderful, compassionate lady. The hospice was also under her direction. Following are excerpts from the little brochure she gave us. Hospices in your area, I am sure, adhere to the same statements of purpose and function.

What Is a Hospice?

"Hospice affirms the basic dignity and worth of life as it serves those who are terminally ill and their families. Crawford County Hospice exists for the purpose of serving those who are terminally ill and their families. We provide hospice care for the physical, emotional and spiritual needs of both the patient and her/his family. The staff of the Hospice will listen, care and understand. We will do all we can to make dying an affirmative part of living."

About three years ago, I could observe that on a closer basis. My one brother-in-law was ill with cancer, and Hospice's nurses took excellent care of him. A wonderful clergyman visited my brother-in-law, and after his passing on, he visited my sister-in-law several times to comfort her and make sure she was all right.

Tribute to a Friendship

The following honors the memory of a woman I have mentioned frequently throughout this book, our support group's treasurer, Jane.

She was my seat neighbor during my first group attendance and the first one to draw me into a conversation.

After becoming an officer, Jane and I quickly became personal friends, visiting and talking on the phone, not only about group matters, but also lots of personal concerns. We talked and joked, griped and complained about life and the people in it, unburdened ourselves and encouraged each other. In short, we talked, we listened, and we lifted each other up.

Two or three months after I, quit she, too, handed in her resignation. We drifted apart for a little while because she and her husband spent the summer camping, and we two only talked occasionally on the phone when she returned to town.

In June of 1996, Jane was hospitalized. On Wednesday, June 19, 1996, she called me, barely able to talk, but she begged me to start thinking more about Elvie than about others, to not carry the burden of the world as she had done for so long. I told her I would ask my husband to bring me down so I could visit with her. We ended the conversation as usual, I exhorting her to hang in, she promising she would because she "hadn't bugged enough people yet," as she always put it.

I had visited with my daughter for a little while on Friday morning, but left her, telling her I wanted to go and see Jane. Well, I wasn't home ten minutes when the phone rang. It was her husband, telling me that she had left us, and he wanted to let me know before I got hit with it at seeing the obituary unawares. Yes, it hurt. It hurt terribly then, and even after eight years, I still miss Jane and her friendship.

On Sunday before Jane's burial, I wrote a little goodbye, and on Monday before the services, I gave it to Bob and asked him if I could put it under her pillow. He instead read it, gave it to the priest and had him read it after Holy Mass. I will reprint it here as a memorial to her and maybe give you an idea for future use, if necessary.

Dearest friend:
  For over the eight years that I have known you, you've tirelessly given of yourself to others. For five years, you

have given your time and energy to the support group. You've served as treasurer, arranged the monthly raffles and the yearly fundraiser picnics, taken care of the literature, helped with addressing cards and the newsletter, called and were called, gave comfort, encouragement and lightened the hearts, minds and souls of those who turned to you.

Jane, in the name of us all, I say, thank you. I also thank you for having been my friend. We've shared tears and laughter, exchanged a little gossip and unburdened ourselves with each other. In short, we were friends, and I thank you for it.

Now you watch us from a better place (yes, you can stop laughing now, Jane), where you no longer have to endure pain or carry the load of others on your shoulders. I'm sad you left us and will miss you, dear friend, but you deserve to rest in God's heavenly peace. As during your life time, I'll continue to think about you, pray for you and love you.

MSWGMD

Why do I tell you all this?

Three reasons. It is a tribute to her memory, the commemoration of a friendship and, I hope, an inspiration for you, should you ever lose a close friend.

A friendship can do so much; it hurts so much when it ends abruptly, and one can't help but thinking, "I should have...Why didn't I...If only...."

But I'm glad I have my memories; I don't feel guilty over having neglected her or used her, and I'm convinced I'll see her again.

MSWGMD

The following selection deals with another subject that may be rejected by some people, it dealing with reincarnation. If you belong to them, please feel free to go on to the next segment.

I think everybody who has MS has asked themselves: "Why? Why me? Why did I have to come down with MS? What have I done to deserve this?"

I have asked these questions too, angry, furious, full of self-pity. I have accused life, heaven, earth and everything in between of having dealt me a lousy hand. And as most people probably are afraid of dying; I, too, feared the end of my life, till I found a new explanation of life and living through belief in reincarnation.

Reincarnation? What's that? Some obscure Eastern religion? Coming back as a stinkweed or skunk? That's only good for horror movies and Gothic books; it surely isn't compatible with Christian beliefs—to which I contend in and love of God or any Higher Being and belief in reincarnation are quite compatible.

My sister-in-law believes in reincarnation, something I had always looked down on in amused pity. In October 1987, I picked up, out of curiosity and to no longer argue from ignorance, the book *Life Between Life* by Whitton and Fisher, an introduction to reincarnation. I struggled against it, but by page thirty-eight, I was hooked, convinced of the validity of the theory and easily embraced the belief. And, surprise to me, after I mentioned it to my husband, he admitted that he believed in reincarnation for a long time.

My reason for the change of mind? You see, I find it comforting to believe that the soul is being reborn in different bodies, that a loving and merciful God gives us more than one chance to get it right, to learn our life lessons, that He gives us His grace, helping us to learn to do what is right, what is pleasing to Him and helping us to become the best person we can be.

Even excluding the MS, my life has not been easy, but I receive comfort from accepting that maybe I have been guilty of some wrongdoings in a previous life, which I want to rectify in this present one. The MS? I have two theories: Maybe I have been unkind to a handicapped person in a previous life, which warrants the hardship of the illness in this one and lets me atone the wrong committed. Or maybe I have chosen to take on the illness to understand it through experiencing on myself what it feels like and share this personal and theoretical knowledge with others. I'm grateful He has also given me a good mind, which makes learning easy and allows me to give something back to others.

The major rewards of believing in reincarnation are these: It grants an incredible peace of mind, soul and spirit. It also grants the relief of knowing that I don't have to accomplish everything in that one setting. In other words, if I goof, I won't be condemned for all eternity.

That does not mean that I'm letting myself get lazy and slack off. I do try to be, become and stay the best person I can possibly be, do the best I can do and hope that will be pleasing to God.

Neither do I want to die; I still have too much to do. But when I'm called, I won't be afraid to go.

And that is something that has greatly helped me gain a different perspective and accept that I have the limitations of multiple sclerosis.

MSWGMD

Now that's definitely enough about me. You now know more about me and my inner world than many people.

This chapter's title says Living, Coping and Accepting. I believe before we can learn to cope with the MS, we have to learn to live with ourselves and the everyday people we come in contact with in our everyday world.

I have coined a phrase for my other non-fiction book, it being *Living in Inner Freedom*. That is, even if we don't have the physical freedom of doing what we would like to do or going where we would like to go, we still can gain the inner freedom of acceptance of ourselves, our station in life and the MS we are being saddled with.

To help with that, I will present a report of the meeting I had put together and presented to our group.

MSWGMD

The president had said, "Okay, can we begin?" the necessary business had been taken care of, handouts had been distributed, and she turned the meeting over to me.

Me? Me? Me? U'huh, me who gets flustered when she's expected to speak without a typed out, prepared and well-rehearsed text. Of course I had it all neatly written out, had rehearsed it out loud, but this occurred before I had completed my self-confidence program; thus I was shaking, and my mouth was straw dry.

Why had I put myself through it then?

Well, I had always asked for somebody to speak on a subject I find extremely important—it being acceptance—and several group members had asked about it too. For some reason, we were unable to find a speaker, and I decided I would put something together. Simple, ain't it? I mean, if something is important to you, you go for it and do it yourself if necessary, right?

Taking all that into consideration, I jumped at it.

Oh, since as secretary I was also responsible for keeping the notes of the meeting, I closed my book, indicating that the meeting was just for us who were present, and as far as I was concerned, everything anybody said was off the record and would stay among us. In other words, nothing anybody said would make the newspapers, not even the newsletter. Only the outline would be printed there.

We had us a darn good and productive meeting. Following is the reprint of what I had prepared, beginning with the handout.

Through Honesty in Self-examination You Can Come Closer to Self-acceptance and MS-acceptance

Introduction

What is MS? MS is multiple sclerosis. It's a depressing disease, a scary one, an unpredictable one. It is lack and loss of control, and it is difficult to live life at the mercy of the iffy, erratic and capricious MS. True MS acceptance can lighten the millstone, but attaining it requires some hard thinking work.

Outline, Questions and Suggestions:
Some hang-ups, strengths and weaknesses

Acceptance
You
Acceptance hindrances
How to go about it and how to do it
We began by shortly discussing the following hang-ups,
strengths and weaknesses

*Do you minimize your strengths and successes?
*Do you maximize what you perceive as your weaknesses
and failures?
*Do you know what you like and dislike?
*Do you accept yourself as the person and personality you
are?
*Do you accept that you have multiple sclerosis?
*How did you feel about yourself before you were
diagnosed as having multiple sclerosis?
*How do you see yourself now?
*Is there a discrepancy?
*If you say yes, why?
*Is there something that makes you angry about having
MS? What is it?
*Do you feel guilty?
*If you say yes, when do you feel guilty? Why do you feel
guilty? About what do you feel guilty?
*What do you fear most about having multiple sclerosis?
*What do you hate most about having multiple sclerosis?
*Do you feel inferior because you have multiple sclerosis?
*Do you feel like damaged merchandise?
*Have you forgiven yourself for having multiple sclerosis?

As I said, we discussed that shortly; then I repeated the title, and we discussed its components.

Honesty: Being honest and open with ourselves without self-deceptions.
Self-evaluation: Without self-deception, becoming aware of what kind of a person/personality we are.

Self-acceptance: Whole-heartedly accepting ourselves as the individual human being we are, with all our good and what we think are our not-so-good sides.

MS-acceptance: Without shame, guilt, self-devaluation or self-pity accepting that we have multiple sclerosis.

True self-acceptance and true MS-acceptance: That's tough. Very tough. Oh, it's easy to say, maybe flippantly or impatiently, "Oh, I've accepted that I have MS," but did you hear the emphasis on say? Isn't it true that what we say sometimes isn't necessarily what we think and feel? In other words, the saying often doesn't reach deep down in the deeper core of our being.

It's easy to deceive oneself, pride oneself on, say, control, martyrdom, mastering and heroics. Or we can fall prey to being overly careful so as not to endanger the condition of our condition. The most beneficial way toward some sort of inner peace is to continually evaluate and reevaluate our attitude. This alertness toward watching and revising our attitude is an ongoing process.

The thinking process can be started anywhere. From experience I can attest that it's best to start with the easiest area, let's say, reviewing something you know you have already accepted, or tackle somewhere where you are a little amused about yourself, what you do and how you do it. Or you may want to find out first what you truly want, like or dislike—that is, wishing for something other than for the MS to go away.

This attempt of finding our inner core is a necessary necessity. You concentrate on you, on what you personally like, dislike or want. Then you consider how much of it you can realistically expect to receive.

Next we tackled self-awareness.

Why is that important?

For several reasons. Let's say people from Group A (remember, the groups of people I have outlined in "Response to the MS Diagnosis") see themselves as bad or MS-damaged merchandise or find themselves being worth less than normal (healthy) people. They act that self-image out and practically beg to be beaten, kicked and punished—and others, reacting to what they see, oblige by beating, kicking and punishing.

Or people from Group B present themselves as larger-than-life gifts of God to all of creation. They invite scorn, pity and ridicule, it at least being doled out behind their back.

Our Group Cers expect pity for their suffering, Group Ders want admiration for enduring their tribulations, while people from Group E want praise for the hard work they do, despite all what fate has heaped on 'em. All three invite sighs of impatience, head shakes or at least eyes rolled ceilingward. As quickly as possible, people run away from them because they get tired of seeing, hearing and smelling the same ole fish.

And those who have given up their feelings of self-worth because they believe MS has robbed them of their values as human being? Do you think they can expect that others have a high opinion of them?

I had noticed that some of the listeners drew back in their chairs, abandoned my text and ad-libbed.

Yes, I know I keep harping on the same subject ,and I've been told that sometimes I come across as cold, unfeeling, appearing as if I were elevating myself as better 'n others, lacking compassion and locking down on or pitying those that aren't as, uh, advanced as I am. That is hundred-percently untrue. I do care, but I have trouble showing it.

And I definitely don't look down on others, but it is true that I've met people—no, not anybody associated with this group—who do the squat-ins and don't feel like getting off their false stances. I do feel compassion for them because I have been there too. But through self-examination, self-awareness, self- and MS-acceptance, I've learned to change a little for the better. I've been awakened to reality, and I wish I could make everybody believe that we all are wonderful human beings. We're imperfect, yes, with ordinary personality assets and liabilities, just because we are human beings. But we have the right to change our thinking about ourselves, gaining self-respect and acting in our best interest, which will help us get rid of some of the resentment grudges, and in turn, we can add layer upon layer of self-acceptance over the dungheap of insecurity.

Well, I suppose that did it, they cackled, some questions and comments were offered, and I returned to the prepared text.

Self-acceptance hindrances: Ask yourself another set of questions; find out if, like most of us, you also tend to maximize what you perceive as flaws, weaknesses and failings, and minimize your strengths, assets and successes because—or so do we believe—we've been nagged at so often that we lack in this and that and those areas, and besides, it's not nice to brag about oneself since there's oh so much wrong with us.

I looked up, grinned and explained: For instance, for the longest time, I had trouble putting in the newsletter and the newspaper write-ups what I had said in group or what I had done for the group because I feared it might sound like bragging. Yep, then I didn't recognize that as low self-worth-feelings or self-putdown. You might have noticed that I've changed that.

We discussed ways toward gaining self-acceptance—asking ourselves what we were good at, using self-observation, stopping to put ourselves down and instead lift ourselves up, admitting that we were better persons than we thought we were—and I proceeded on to MS-acceptance.

After we have learned to accept ourselves, after we've gained practice in seeing things realistically—that is, seeing them as they are and not as we want them to be, not as we think they are or as they ought, should or must be or as others tell us they are—we can tackle the MS-acceptance. We can cool-mindedly assess MS, what it is, what it truly does to us, what it prevents us from doing. We can learn to put it in its rightful place, giving it neither a too high nor too low a priority ranking and take back at least some of the power we have handed over to it.

Here are a few mind-joggers to start your considerations with: Multiple sclerosis is an imperfection of the body. Some people have ulcers, others have allergies, and some have smelly feet. Do they tell themselves they're worth less because of this? Not very likely, huh.

It won't help the disposition of our disposition if we accuse heaven, earth, hell and everything in between that life has dealt us a lousy hand. That not only raises our blood pressure, but it also pounds down on the immune system—and we know neither of these two stresses is good for us. If we calmly accept facts factually—okay, okay, if we as calmly as possible accept facts factually—we have a better chance of feeling better, feel less stressed, and that lessens, shortens and soothes exacerbations.

After you have worked through these steps, you can face the questions from the outline, answer them in a more factual frame of mind and try, over and over if necessary, accepting that you have multiple sclerosis.

One very important question to assess is the one about how you felt about yourself before and after your diagnosis. If there is a major discrepancy, especially a marked drop in the self-esteem area, please do yourself a favor and try getting that self-esteem level back to where it belongs—at least to pre-diagnosis levels.

Another good question to ponder is the one asking whether it makes you angry that you have MS. If your answer is yes or yes, darn it, or even howl a resounding yes, damn it, and I don't like it, and it makes me angry, congratulations! It shows that you're a fighter and won't allow MS to get you down. And I do believe righteous anger also stimulates endorphin production.

Yes, you can do it all. You can turn negative feelings into positive affirmations about yourself. You might have multiple sclerosis, but you are also strong, can do battle and fight instead of letting it get you down.

Incidentally, a few more words about negative feelings-unproductive anger, that is, anger which doesn't lead to change but to fear, guilt, self-pitying, giving up-don't push them out of your mind. You might manage not to think about them consciously but believe me, they're not out of mind because they are out of sight. Like The Factor X trigger, who never rests but continues to think up new tricks to aggravate us, so do negative feelings continue to do their dirty work. Thus for your own good, face up to those buggers as calmly as you can, accept them as legitimate because they come out of your mind and till you get rid of them through realistic thinking they are part of you. After accepting that premise, you can stretch yourself to your full mental health, realize how unrealistic they are, come to grips with them and get rid of them.

As with all mental processes, the fight for acceptance is an on-going procedure. New hindrances creep up. As soon as we have one of the old ones licked a new one creeps up or one of the real old ones reappears. But I can tell you from experience, with time it gets easier to spot'm and head'm off at the pass.

Self-discovery brings the potential of shame. While digging through the rubble of years of people-pleasing, low-self-esteem-holding, one-upmanship, self-deceptions, competing against others, comparing ourselves to others and finding ourselves lacking, elevating ourselves and putting others down or vice versa, we might be unable to believe that we could have any reason to believe in ourselves or hold ourselves in high esteem. It is a common practice that people try to get rid of that pain be resorting to lying to themselves; that is, slipping into self-deceptions. But we won't let that sidetrack us for too long; we are fighters.

When you do uncover your real Self, wow, will you be pleasantly surprised at finding the great person you are. And with that, you can finally accept yourself as you are.

I have heard vociferous objections, telling me that that changing sounds too much like work.

So? Doesn't achieving anything worthwhile deserves an honest effort? But, hey, the benefits will be well worth any of the energy expended.

Now let me give you my bottom line:

I have accepted that I am not perfect and need not be perfect. All that is required of me is that I do the best I can do and be the best person I can be. I accept that I am an imperfect individual person and that striving for perfection could be more damaging to my health than my smoking.

How Can We Help?

That is a question I heard and still hear from family, friends, acquaintances and community members. My answer is this:

Treat us like the normal human beings we are, even if we can't walk as fast, think as fast, talk as fast as you do. Don't scare us with horror stories. Inform yourself, or ask us, about the facts of what multiple sclerosis is and what it does to us.

When we are in the dumps, yes, we would appreciate a kind word, bolstering our spirits, comforting us and giving us a little support, especially when we're in the dumps, maybe even receiving some unasked-for help. Some say a hug would do heaps of good.

What to avoid: Don't baby us; don't overdo the doing for us. Let us handle what we are able to handle ourselves. Don't demand we do things your way or don't do certain other things. We may be ill in body, but in most cases, our minds work quite well. Please don't talk down to us as if we were helpless little kids who don't know what's good or bad for them. Don't speak for us. Unless our speech is totally unhearable or ununderstandable, we can communicate what is on our mind or respond to questions with pertinent answers. So ask us, not the person who may accompany us. We are quite able to think logically.

MSWGMD

I must say a few words about the town I have called home since 1975.

Galion is inhabited by friendly people who care for and about us who don't get around too well. I have already told you about my experience at the used book sale. When I and my walker or cane go to a store, people hold the door open, and many say a kind word. Yes, school kids and teenagers in Galion do that, too. Of course I say, "Thank you; I appreciate it," with an open smile and an expression that shows that I mean it.

My daughter and her family, her computer whizzzz husband, her musician and computer whizzz son and risk-taking young son live just across the street from me. This street is part of the town's main thoroughfare and, at times, quite busy. Well, most of the cars coming from either direction have stopped and let me cross, no matter how long the line of cars behind them was. Even the patrolman in one of the police cruisers stopped and let me cross instead of citing me for jaywalking.

Yes, I appreciate the Galionites' kindness; I like living in this town and will resist any nudge toward moving anywhere else.

(I have copied these last three paragraphs and submitted them on 7 May 2002 as a Letter to the Editor for our *Galion Inquirer*, to let Galionites know that their courtesy is appreciated.)

Chapter Six
Some Encouragements

I want to end our talk with some encouragement pieces I have written in past and present times.

Coping with multiple sclerosis isn't easy. It can bring a person to her or his knees—and not only in prayer—but acceptance can lighten the load and helps with the coping. No matter how severely you are struck, you are still the master of your soul, mind and spirit, and most of us are, at least to a partial degree, masters over our lives. Our beliefs about ourselves in particular and our life in general, our assumptions and attitudes, they provide us with at least a semblance of control and self-determination. It all depends on our view whether we want to self-pityingly feel lousy and sorry for ourselves or if we are so busy with living that we don't have time to give in to that darned MS. (Feel free to use stronger language; I do.)

Yes, even if our energy level is at its lowest, when we feel we can't or don't want to make another move, even if we feel totally given out, there are still things we can do.

MSWGMD

Let me tell you how I spell "Coping with Multiple Sclerosis":

C: Care for yourself with courtesy, kindness and respect.
O: Oh yes, you may have MS, but you are still you, a wonderful, unique, worthwhile individual human being, created in God's image.
P: Past, present and future—put them all in the right perspective.
I: In your own best interest, gently let go of your fears.
N: Negative feelings—like giving up because we have multiple sclerosis—renounce them soundly.
G: Go for it; go get it; go on

W: While you're at it, renew your belief in yourself.
I: Immensely important: Thinking determines how you feel, so do a lot of it and live as fully as possible—and not thinking life is full of you-know-what.
T: Trip up depressive feelings with looking for the pretty things in life.
H: Help yourself as much as you can and let God and others do the rest.

M: Moaning and groaning without action-taking is wasteful.
U: Ultimately you are responsible for your life; make the best of it.
L: Love yourself; you're worth it.
T: Tolerance—show it to yourself and others.
I: Irregardless of what life hands you, don't give up on it or on yourself.
P: Put in your fair share of living.
L: Luck doesn't just happen; you have to create it yourself.
E: Errors we learn something from aren't errors; they are lessons learned.

S: Strength gives courage; courage gives strength.
C: Come on; you can do more than you think.
L: Let go of feeling sorry for yourself.
E: Energetically tackle your problems, and you come closer to winning the battle.
R: Rise above the limits MS tries to impose on you .

O: Options are available; you find them if you diligently search for them.

S: Some days are worse than others; make the best of them anyway.

I: If necessary, do some rigorous mental housecleaning.

S: Stay in charge of your life and everything happening in it.

MSWGMD

Just before I put the Christmas newsletter together, I received a letter from a troubled group member and decided to print it with my answers to her as my Christmas present to all. Following is the text, modified as everything else in this edition.

Q. What do you do on bad days?

A. When I'm badly in the dumps and think life is no longer worth to be lived, when I'm deeply dispirited, I give in to self-pity, depression and despair. Maybe I'll curse everything I can think of for a little while—half a day maximum. Or if it concerns a soulwish—that is, something that is very important to me—and I don't receive it, I might take a whole day and night.

But eventually I think the situation through, evaluate it realistically and force myself to do something, anything, mostly routine stuff like doing the laundry, dusting, cooking, putting a cake together. I might even scrub the cabinets. It hasn't been bad enough yet to attack the stove. In fact, my daughter told me she can tell when I'm depressed because then I'm working in and around the kitchen.

At other times, I write one heck of a nasty letter to life, fate, destiny, what or whomever I can think of. (Yes, sometimes I even write one to God, though to Him I'm not nasty, just honest about how I feel.) After I read that composition, though, maybe a couple of hours later when I feel more upbeat, I can grin a little sheepish and bury it in the wet garbage.

Q. What thoughts calm your worst fears?

A. I give myself a good talking to. Not mean or nasty or contemptuous, just something like, "Okay, Elvira, come on; that's enough. Worry won't get you anywhere; it only makes things worse and exaggerates reality. So keep on living in the here and now; enjoy life as it is. Remember, life is something like the Ohio weather; if you don't like it don't worry, it'll change in five minutes."

I also tend to hum my fight song, if necessary through clenched teeth or tear-watered eyes, about not giving up and not letting life flatten me. There are also a couple of German hit tunes that give me encouragement. One of them, my favorite, was popular in the early fifties and goes, translated, something like this:

> Everything will be all right again.
> Just keep your faith and courage
> Even when happiness leaves you for a while.
> As (the month of) May always follows April,
> So will your suffering be replaced by joy
> And you needn't be so sad any longer.
> The sun can't shine every day.
> Those who laugh must occasionally cry.
> But everything will be all right again.
> Just keep your faith and courage.

Q. Where do you find that extra helping of strength and courage when you think everything you have is lost?

A. I have a few inspirational books that I have near my chair for just such an occasions. I open one of them at random and let the words soothe me. Otherwise I try to improvise on the above questions, telling myself that this too shall pass. (As a matter of fact, I have found a perpetual calendar with exactly this title—This Too Shall Pass. Otherwise I listen to soothing music, mostly Mozart. I used to go to my old records and tapes from the fifties and sixties, but found they increased the melancholic sadness. I also go to the bulletin boards, read the postings, some of which mirror my personal concerns, or I vent, as it is being called. You know, talking about how one feels.)

Q. How do you deal with depression?
A. With a lot of thinking and talking to myself. I've said it in a previous newsletter (and will reprint that here) severe and long-lasting depression has to be brought to a qualified health professional, but the minor depressive feelings of shorter duration and severity I deal with myself.

To begin with, I check superficially if I'm angry at somebody and have turned it inward, against myself, as for instance, say that I may have been angry at somebody I'm supposed to love, like a parent, spouse or child, while my mind chides me that it's not nice to be angry. (I say superficially because I do not believe that anger turned inward is the major cause for depression.)

Then I check if I have lost something or fear losing it, be that something tangible (like a piece of jewelry, one of my house plants or my house itself, which was a realistic fear for me a few months ago after my husband died and my financial situation looked bleak) or something intangible (like love, a friendship, a loved one being ill). I also check carefully if I have violated a should (have I done something my insides told me I should not do, or have I not done something I had been told by my oughts, should'ves and musts that I had to do). Repressing guilt, anxiety or fear can also bring on depressive feeling.

If I find a concrete cause for the depression, I analyze it and deal with it the way I deal with fears; I look at the root, assess the reality content of the emotion, reassure myself, and knowing what goes on, I can let it go.

Otherwise I, as the saying goes, just go with the flow. I try not to dwell on it but keep busy and wait for it to subside.

I frequently hear or read about an MS-depression connection, although neither literature has said anything specific, whether depression is a byproduct of MS symptoms or whether the MS itself causes the depression. Maybe it's just the limits of the symptoms that send us in that melancholy? Or is it the chemical imbalance? I don't know. I'm just glad my neurologist has talked me into taking the anti-depressant.

Her last question though really got to me.

Q. What do you do when the soul is as dry as the desert?
A. I turn on my fiber-optic lamp, put my music on—Mozart mainly at such times—lean my head against the back of the chair or the pillow on the bed and let the music and the soft, changing lights drip inner peace back into my soul.
    Of course a little talk with God does also help.

MSWGMD

I also want to share with you my "ABC for Living and Coping With MS." I wrote it for newsletter #12, and it was reprinted in *Relay*.

A. I'm able to share my troubles, burdens and hardships with somebody and help others to carry their load.
B. Be a fighter.
C. Courage will help me through the worst exacerbation.
D. Depression is nothing to be ashamed of; after all, it's difficult to never know what will happen when.
E. Everybody needs somebody to lean onto sometimes.
F. Flip my lid? Only of it helps me getting rid of that mental junk that bugs the H-E-double toothpicks outta me.
G. Giving up? Ha, no me. Giving in? Double ha!!!

H. Helpful people are a God-send; I'm not too proud to reach for and grasp the hand held out to me.

I. I have multiple sclerosis, but it doesn't have me.

J. Joking to laughter feeling better forgetting at least for a little while the bumps and grinds of having multiple sclerosis.

K. Keep your chin up.

L. Letting MS getting the upper hand? Over me and my life? Fattest of chances.

M. MS won't succeed in invoking self-pity in me.

N. Nothing can take away my feeling of being a worthwhile individual, even if I have MS.

O. Over-doing, doing too much, not doing enough, is not a sign of strength but signifies put-downish insecurity. I avoid any of that.

P. People who pity themselves are poor indeed.

Q. Questions like "Why me?" won't do much for my disposition; I'll eliminate them from my vocabulary and ask instead: "What can I still do?"

R. Reality-focus helps me accept the world as it is; I won't expect too much, nor will I be satisfied with too little.

S. I stay in control; if my body doesn't allow me much freedom of movement I'm still in control of my mind.

T. "Think positive" may be a platitude, but why reject it if it is helpful?

U. Under no circumstances will I permit a defeatist attitude to make me lose out on anything life has to offer me.

V. Vigilantly I am on the look-out to prevent my being victimized by MS.

W. Winners don't give up. I'm a winner in life's game plan and won't give up fighting, hoping and living.

X. "X" stands for the unknown which is MS; I cope with it as best as I can.

Y. Yes, MS is hard to live with, but I belong to an elite group of people who master the tough life.

Z. I zero in on my strengths instead of on my weaknesses,
and with God's help, I will be the best person I can be.

My Seven Point Plan for Coping with MS

1. I accept that I am me, accept all my good and not-so-good sides, accept myself as the individual person and personality I am.

2. I accept that thinking plays a major role in my life, that it determines how I feel about myself, my world, my life and the people in it.

3. I accept that I have multiple sclerosis.

4. I accept that I have limits, and I live within these limits.

5. I accept that I need the help of people and things—family, friends, doctors, medications, cane, walker and in the future possibly a wheelchair—to allow me to stay as mobile, productive and independent as possible.

6. I accept that I can no longer do all the things I used to do, liked to do, enjoyed doing, even things I merely had to do. I accept all that, not shouting with glee, but I do accept it.

7. I accept that I need to observe my actions, reactions and interactions, that I need to keep a hold on my impressions of life and what happens in it, that I need to work consciously on my interpretations of these events, and that I have to keep my mood and attitude under my personal control, not under the control of negative feelings like useless, pain-hiding anger, fears, self-putdowns, self-deceptions, self-doubts, deceiving myself or others about my physical and psychological status.

In short, I accept myself as I am; I accept my life as it is; I accept the people in it as they are.

MSWGMD

In 1966, before my family and I left Germany for the United States, my sister gave me a candle with a little poem printed on it. Over the years, I have used it as basis for courage and encouragement. I want to give it to you and end this book with a translation of it:

Whenever you're defeated and feel you can't go on,
Comes from somewhere a little light.
Welcome it, let it in, it will help you
Conquer life just once more
And you can sing of sunshine and joy again,
This little light, it helps you carry your burden
And makes it easier to gain back your courage, strength
and belief.

I have added:

This little light, if you let it into your life,
If you let it light your way
If you allow it, it will give you the strength
To refuse to give up
And you won't let MS get you down.

The End

Appendix A

As I have mentioned earlier, I have written several Letters to the Editor of the *Galion Inquirer*, 378 N. Market Street, Galion, OH 44833. Several of them exceeded the length specifications, but they printed them uncut. As I said, I really thank them for helping me getting the message out.

Once again I wish to stress that I don't want to brag about what I have done. I just want to give you an idea what can be done.

Following is letter number one, printed in the *Galion Inquirer*. I'm sorry, but on this one I have forgotten to put the date notation on. These letters are reprinted unchanged from the originals—although nowadays I would change, add and subtract.

> I have been active in the 1992 nationwide drive to request the Food and Drug Administration grant speedy approval of Beta Interferon as the first drug specifically geared toward treatment of multiple sclerosis. I have learned the FDA was overwhelmed with petitions and they actually did act speedily. I have also received reports of nine pharmaceutical houses who work on developing medications specifically designed to help MS patients.
>
> BUT THINGS ARE NOT MOVING. Following are, as I see it, the major roadblocks:

1. The National MS Society funds research which is designed to prove their theories, viewpoints and standpoints. They have shifted their priorities and spend less money on pure research. I haven't heard much about any lobbying efforts of theirs or their trying to put MS before the public. (I wonder what their admin costs are.)

2. Since MS affects such a relatively small percentage of people (the numbers have been finally upgraded to 450,000 individuals in the US suffering from this disease) researchers feel justified to concentrate on illnesses which are more in the public limelight and thus bring the potential of public acclaim. Pharmaceutical houses, even though they receive help through the Orphan Drug Act, concentrate on the more profitable drugs for the many. Many diseases have powerful and vocal spokespersons. The government and governmental agencies give the loudmouths more of what they want and lawmakers grant the well-known diseases money because more people who vote are affected by the disease.

3. Multiple sclerosis patients are too silent, too timid, too laid back. They don't make waves, just take it, don't stand up for themselves and their rights. Too many are still too scared of being shunned or, as somebody told me, being dropped by their insurance company if they have a chronic disease.

Isn't it time that we people who have MS, with the help of our families, friends and other concerned people, make our voices heard and demand that we're being listened to and treated fairly? We and our families pay taxes, we vote, we deserve our fair share of attention, research time and money. Let's demand it. Not ask for it—demand it.

As I said in my personal letter writing campaign (I sent out fifty two letters) I realize AIDS is a terrible disease and deserves the resources necessary to combat it. But is it fair to commit all money, research and time to AIDS and underfund or overlook other diseases which make people sick and cause suffering for patients and their families?

We people who are at the mercy of multiple sclerosis would appreciate any help anybody could give us. Remember the squeaky wheel which gets oiled?

To all MSers, best wishes for permanent remission, Elvira K. (Elvie) James.

MSWGMD

Below is letter number two, printed by the *Inquirer* around October 15, 1994:

I wish to thank the staff of the Galion Inquirer for keeping their editorial eyes open and report on the meager news about multiple sclerosis, (a disease) which is still quite prevalent in our town.

I outlined the story and history of copolymer-1 and continued with:

...tout it as a brand new discovery—which, of course requires extensive, expensive and lengthy testing to satisfy the FDA which will cost exorbitant sums which will make it near—impossible for the patient who has to count quarters instead of hundred dollar bills to obtain the medication when it finally hits the markets in half a dozen or more years at starkly inflated prices.

Just look at Betaseron. It costs $10,000 (that was in 1996) for a year's supply. I ask: Is that a realistic cost? How much of this is recuperating the cost of research, testing and paperwork to satisfy the FDA? How much of it is profit for the pharmaceutical house? How much is the government subsidy from the Orphan Drug Act? Is this give-away used to reduce the price of the drug?

I agree, our medication should be tested and proven safe for human consumption but what the dictators at the FDA demand goes beyond the boundaries of the reasonable. And don't forget the drugs which are kept from the market, drugs which were tested, proven effective and used for many years in other countries, copolymer-1 for instance had its origin in Israel. I never found out how far the testing went and/or if it had been prescribed for Israeli MSers. Could it be that the FDA oppressors insist on extensive re-testing—well, see paragraph and question above.

Yes, I'm angry and bitter.

To all MSers, best wishes for permanent remission.

To tell you the truth, I had feared they'd clean it up, but nope, they printed it fully as I had typed it. They're great people, the editorial staff at the *Galion Inquirer*.

MSWGMD

Here is number three, printed in the *Inquirer* on April 11, 1995:

I was extremely saddened by the story in the *Galion Inquirer* of 6 April 1995. A woman, diagnosed with multiple sclerosis, felt compelled by fear of the illness, to kill herself and her mother who depended on her care.

In addition to sadness, I also felt helpless anger that MS still evokes such terror in people stricken with MS, a fear which, in my opinion, is caused by misinformation and lack of factual information.

Yes, a small percentage of people are hit by the chronic-progressive type of MS and their symptoms develop faster and cause a more severe course of suffering. But most MSers are afflicted less severely. They can't perform certain activities they had formerly taken for granted or they now perform them less efficiently because of certain impairments, but they are still contributing members of family, community and society.

Many MSers I know fall into this category; they hold full time jobs, they are fathers or mothers who raise their children or as homemakers or self-employed persons provide a needed service.

I wrote a few sentences about my personal experiences and ended with this paragraph:

In summary I'd like to say this: Becoming informed about MS takes some of the fear of the unpredictability of the disease away, gives the strength of acceptance, helps with coping with the impairments (and grants the ingenuity) to devise adaptive strategies and leads to not giving up in despair or giving in to self-pitying laying down and giving up.

MSWGMD

Following is part of the open letter I composed and sent to area doctors, hospitals, physical and occupational therapy departments with the request to guide their patience to us:

Hi.

Like you, we have MS. We're not glad that you have joined our ranks but you can believe us, the diagnosis nor the illness are neither the end of the world nor the end of your life. You may be devastates by fears, you may think life is no longer worth to be lived, you may even doubt your worth and value as a human being but that is not true. It's not true at all.

We won't say: I know how you feel. Nobody can do that but we do feel with you-the diagnosis as well as living with MS is frightening.

But right now we have the advantage of belonging to a multiple sclerosis support group. I say with confidence that 98.765 percent of people will be comfortable belonging to our group. We are informal, charge no dues, we laugh together, are serious together and simply try to do what our name indicates-we try to give support to each other and accept support from others.

What can you expect from us?

The following paragraph outlined what I have already told you—giving addresses, phone numbers, meeting time and place, the newsletter, availability of literature and continued:

If you'd like to attend our meetings, we'll be glad to welcome you and will try to make you comfortable. If you want to talk we'll try to answer as best as we can. If you prefer to stay silent, we'll respect that too. If you just want the introductory package, we'll send it to you in a plain envelope. If you just want to receive the newsletter we'll gladly add you to our mailing list and you can rest assured that nobody will see it.

We're not out to boost our membership numbers, we believe we can offer you comfort, answer questions because we understand that coping with multiple sclerosis makes for a very difficult life—and that is putting it mildly.

A short official introduction with phone numbers, as well as meeting time and place as well as handicapped accessibility and parking notes ended the letter.

MSWGMD

I had planned to copy the letter my daughter ,and I sent to lawmakers, political candidates, TV and radio stations, but after rereading it I realized that everything I said in it has already been said. I'm sure you can put something personal together from what I have presented.

I just want to say to all MS person who read this: Best wishes for permanent remission

—Elvie

Printed in the United States
48928LVS00005B/253-267